Looking Through the Window at Dementia

The Caregiver's Handbook to Understanding Dementia

By Laura Banner, Certified Family Nurse Practitioner

TABLE OF CONTENTS

Dedication

This book is dedicated to:

All those who have graciously entrusted me with the care of their loved one.

My mom Sandy. When I think about the love and support Mom has given unconditionally every single day of my life, I am humbled...and incredibly thankful. As a single parent, she sacrificed for me in ways that I will never be able to fully comprehend. Nor will I ever be able to adequately express my appreciation and admiration for all she has done, other than to say, "I love you".

My husband Bob. You are my loving husband and best friend. When I met and married you, my world was forever changed. You make me smile like no other, laugh like I've never laughed and love like I never thought possible. You are my dream come true. Thank you for believing in me and encouraging me to chase my dreams. I love you now and forever!

Introduction

According to the National Alzheimer's Association…

- One in three seniors is suffering from some form of dementia when they die.
- Alzheimer's is the 6th leading cause of death in the United States.
- More people die from some form of dementia than from breast cancer and prostate cancer *combined*.
- More than 16 million Americans are providing care to a loved one with some form of dementia without getting paid.
- Almost 1/3 of these caregivers is over the age of 65.
- Most volunteer caregivers are daughters of the patient.
- These volunteer caregivers are giving almost 19 BILLION hours of care each year.
- The number of seniors with dementia is expected to nearly triple over the next thirty years; rising from 5 million (now) to 14 million.

The facts and figures aren't pleasant to think about but refusing to see the reality of the situation only makes a sad and difficult situation sadder and more difficult. The possibility that you will find yourself caring for a loved one with dementia is real. So is the possibility that you will *be* the one with dementia. This is not meant a message of doom and gloom. It is more like a call to arms to prepare…just in case.

It is far better to have what you need and not need it, than to need what you don't have. In this case, the 'need' is knowledge and information. Specifically, knowledge and information on how to care for someone with dementia—what to expect, where to go for help, what to do, and what not to do.

Providing this type of information and support is the reason I founded **Compassionate Education, LLC**. The mission of Compassionate Education is to provide accurate and useful information to families and caregivers about dementia while instilling confidence in the caregiver.

This book is a byproduct of my practice. It is a collection of the most often-asked questions and concerns of caregivers—both those I meet with and those who reach out to me via my podcast and blog.

It is my privilege and honor to offer this book to you as a resource of information and encouragement as you take a difficult but rewarding journey.

-Laura

Foreword

The Hippocratic Oath is the promise every doctor makes to care for their patients to the best of their ability. But doctors know they cannot do it alone. They know it takes a village of healthcare workers to be able to give patients the quality of care and quantity of attention they need. This is especially true for patients with dementia.

General practitioners and specialists alike recognize the value of working alongside caregivers like Laura to provide patients and their families the best possible care and attention. The following votes of confidence from two highly respected neurologists are proof of that.

"By 2030 all baby boomers will have reached age 65. This graying of America, as it is being called, brings with it associated age-related illnesses, including dementia. As a neurologist, I diagnose and treat a large number of dementia patients and their families. Sadly, the time I spend with them is meager compared to the time they need. Laura Banner's compassionate and dignified methods of caring for dementia patients and their families is filling that gap for many who find themselves navigating the confusing, frightening, and (at times) comical waters of dementia."

"Laura's book is educational and entertaining—an absolute 'must read'!"

-Shaena Blevins, MD

"I have worked with Laura professionally for nearly ten years, and I am honored that she asked me to write a few words for her book. I continue to be inspired by her unwavering passion for patients and families suffering from degenerative cognitive disorders. She has shown an uncanny ability and depth of knowledge which has proven to be an indispensable asset within our neurology service.

-Jonathan Kerrick, MD

An Introduction to Dementia

As a career state law enforcement officer, I knew the possibility existed that I would have to move my family to a different part of the state in order to rise through the ranks, i.e. get promoted. Not a lot, but once or twice over the course of twenty-five to thirty years was not unusual.

That time came two years after my grandpa died. That fact is relevant because my wife, three small children, and I lived less than a mile from them—now just my grandma. The grandma whose yard we mowed, the grandma who loved on and played with our children several times a week, the grandma our children adored, the grandma whose car and house I kept in tip-top shape, and so on and so on. In other words, it was a big decision to make, but in the end, we left, because leaving meant we would also be able to take over my wife's family farm. Besides, we could come back when we wanted and when things needed my attention. It was only a three-hour drive.

For the first year, things went smoothly. We made a few trips back and Grandma even came to spend a few days with us a couple of times (thanks to some friends who were able to help with transportation). But then one evening I got a phone call from one of our best friends who was also the preacher at our church—the church Grandma had been a member of since before I was born.

He said he'd been to visit Grandma that day 'just because', but that she was not herself. He went on to tell us that she talked about having spent the previous evening visiting with several people (she called them by name). The problem was that every single one of those people had been dead for

1

several years. After that, we started getting other calls and notes from friends back home voicing similar concerns. We noticed these things ourselves when we visited a few weekends later, but no matter how we tried to approach it, she became either defensive or hurt.

A few months and several incidents later, we finally had to move Grandma into an assisted living facility. As part of the process, she underwent a thorough examination that included several different tests. The doctor's explanation of Grandma's dementia was this: "Her brain is short circuiting. And as time goes on, the circuits become more frayed and fragile until they quit working altogether. Now I know that's far from being the most accurate medical explanation of what happens to someone with dementia, but for me, it was the type of word picture I could relate to. It helped put things into perspective, helped alleviate the frustration and guilt I was feeling, and allowed me to be at peace with the decision to move her out of her home into a place she could be watched over and cared for. ~John

John is right in saying that the doctor's word picture isn't very medical-esque, but I have to admit it is an acceptable way to explain with simplistic accuracy. Keeping things simple without sacrificing facts and accuracy is important when explaining dementia to a patient and/or their family and caregivers.

Equally important, is explaining what dementia is not, because of all the misconceptions, misunderstanding, and misinformation surrounding this awful disease.

Are you a caregiver to someone with dementia, or maybe a family member of someone with dementia? Or are you worried that maybe sometime in the future you might develop this awful disease? If so, then you will undoubtedly find the following facts and information about dementia highly informative and helpful.

The first thing you should know is that dementia is not a diagnosis, it is a medical term. It is the umbrella term used in and out of the medical profession used to describe abnormal/organic memory loss.

Now, before we even take another breath, let's clarify what constitutes abnormal/organic memory loss. Abnormal or organic memory loss is memory loss that cannot be attributed to medication, fatigue, depression, or some other cause such as a concussion, high fever, or extreme illness. And to add to that, you need to know that abnormal/organic memory loss is memory loss that does not improve once you address and treat the issue or root cause of the memory loss.

First let's look at normal memory loss. This is also often referred to as age-related memory loss. People often confuse normal memory loss with dementia, but it's not the same thing.

Dementia isn't filling in the blank where the date goes with the wrong date. Dementia isn't forgetting we put the keys to the car or the house in our pocket instead of the basket on the kitchen counter like we always do. Dementia isn't forgetting one of you grandchild's middle name or getting their birthdays mixed up. Those things are age-related memory loss. They are just part of life and don't really have any effect on the quality of your life. They are merely annoyances and inconveniences. That's all.

Dementia, on the other hand, is quite different. Instead of putting the keys in your pocket, you put them in the refrigerator or the oven. Or in many cases, you forget what they are used for. You don't just forget your grandchild's middle name. It's forgetting that person is your grandchild. See the difference?

So once again, before we move on to the facts about dementia, while the normal age-related memory loss is bothersome, it is wise to be aware of it and acknowledge it, because it will make it easier for you and your loved ones to recognize and deal with more serious memory loss should it occur.

Now for what dementia is...

The term dementia is most often paired with Alzheimer's, when in fact, Alzheimer's disease is just one type of dementia. The most common forms of dementia besides Alzheimer's include:

•Vascular dementia: dementia caused by a lack of blood flow and oxygen to the brain.

•Dementia associated with Lewy Body: dementia caused by excess protein deposits on the brains' nerve cells.

•Parkinson's-related dementia: dementia that is part of the progression of Parkinson's disease.

•Multi-infarct dementia: dementia that results when someone who has had multiple strokes that take a toll on their memory and their thought process

•Alcohol-related dementia: dementia caused by the erosion and destruction of the brain cells due to alcoholism.

•Frontotemporal dementia: the term used to describe a dementia in which proteins clump and accumulate in frontal and temporal lobes of the brain ultimately impair those areas in the brain from working properly. It can also be the result of injury or illness that adversely affects the frontal and temporal lobes of the brain.

Granted, Alzheimer's is by far the most prevalent form of dementia. In fact, two-thirds of all people with some type of dementia, either have Alzheimer's or what we call 'mixed dementia', which is a combination of (usually) Alzheimer's and some other form of dementia.

Mixed dementias are actually becoming more and more common than they used to be. Whether that is because we didn't realize what we were actually dealing with before, or because more people are being affected by different catalysts for dementia is unclear. Either way, however, the fact remains that we are seeing more mixed dementia than we used to.

For example, someone will initially present one type of dementia—perhaps vascular dementia. As time goes on, however, they start presenting symptoms of another type of dementia such as Alzheimer's. So, instead of using the term vascular dementia and Alzheimer's dementia, we just combine it, and we refer to two or more types of dementia as mixed dementia.

When talking about Alzheimer's we need to realize that there is more than one kind of Alzheimer's disease. First on the list is early-onset Alzheimer's, which is Alzheimer's that initially presents itself in people under the age of sixty-five.

The other type of Alzheimer's is late-onset Alzheimer's, which is Alzheimer's that presents symptoms in people age sixty-five or older.

The medical community admits there is still much to learn about dementia. But we are also able to say that over the past several years, we have made enormous strides in recognizing dementia, slowing down the progression (in many cases, but not all), and in making resources available to both patients and caregivers that increases the quality of life for everyone involved.

For example, we know is that when someone has early-onset Alzheimer's, they tend to progress through the stages of the disease much quicker than someone who has late-onset Alzheimer's. Therefore, if someone develops Alzheimer's or some other form of memory loss (dementia) when they are eighty-five years old, and another individual develops the same or similar impairment, at age, sixty, in five years, the person who was sixty (now sixty-five) will be much further down the road in terms of cognitive decline that the person who was 85 (now 90).

Looking at it from that perspective, this is actually one of those times when age is on your side. The older you are at onset of symptoms, the slower the disease tends to progress, which for the patient, is actually digression.

NOTE: early and late-onset Alzheimer's is not to be confused or interchanged with early and late stages of Alzheimer's. Stages refers to the progression of the disease rather than the age of the patient at the time of diagnosis.

Because Alzheimer's is the leading form of dementia, I also want to share some important facts with you about this dreadful, awful disease. My reason for doing so is to make you more aware of the need for ongoing research, and equally important (if not more so), to make you aware of the need for you to be watchful, aware, and proactive in caring for yourself or your loved ones should you or they be stricken with Alzheimer's, or any other form of dementia, for that matter.

Did you know that:

•Alzheimer's is the sixth leading cause of death in the United States?

•That Alzheimer's is responsible for more deaths than breast cancer and prostate cancer combined?

•That people have regular wellness screens for breast and prostate cancer, but very few people bother with wellness screenings for Alzheimer's or other forms of dementia?

The lack of wellness screenings is puzzling to me, especially since the vast majority of seniors believe memory screenings and evaluations are incredibly important. Unfortunately, when they go for their annual wellness checks, most are not being asked about memory issues.

This needs to change. Whether you are a senior, or still in your 20s 30s or 40s, you need to be thinking about this. You need to know that you have a 66% chance that dementia will directly impact your life at some point.

Or maybe that point is now—maybe your life is already being affected. Maybe you're the one with the memory issue. Maybe your parent or spouse has dementia and maybe you are the caregiver. You might even be part of the sandwich generation—taking care of your parents while still raising your children. Chances are also good that you are still working and trying to balance it all without letting anyone feel like a burden. Yet you are struggling to keep it together.

The best piece of advice I have for both individuals and family members facing the onslaught of dementia can be summed up in one word: PROACTIVE.

By being proactive, you can save yourself and your family from serious heartache and stress. By being proactive, you can prevent serious errors in judgement and decision-making from being made.

Things like errors in taking (or not) their medication, financial decisions, bill paying, and so forth. Remember that these aren't just personal issues. These are issues that affect one's safety. Families need to get involved. They need to have conversations, because the earlier the diagnosis, the easier (less controversial) these conversations will be. Not that they are ever easy, as in pleasant or matter of fact but easy from the standpoint that the patient is able to have a say and take ownership in their life and their future.

I understand that these conversations and decisions are bittersweet because unfortunately, at this point we don't have a cure. We have treatments to help reduce and manage symptoms, but we can't stop the progression of the disease. We can't even reverse the progression of the disease. We can only try to manage the symptoms and delay them. But the earlier your loved one is diagnosed, the sooner they can start getting treatment. The sooner they can start participating in future healthcare decisions that will ultimately impact them. So please don't put it off. The longer you wait, the harder it will be—especially when trying to convince someone with dementia that they need your help and intervention.

Unfortunately for me, dementia seems to be woven into the DNA on both sides of my family. We have several family members who have mixed forms of dementia. Because of this, I cannot help but be somewhat frightened. I fear that someday, I too might develop some type of dementia.

My mom lives with me, and she's starting to have some difficulty with word-finding and following along as we tell a story. She gets a little confused with the sequencing of events. It's enough of an issue that I am concerned about it.

So is she. And even though, in my professional role, I diagnose and treat dementia patients every day, when it hits that close to home, I'm no different than you are. I try to dismiss Mom's actions by passing them off as fatigue or mild depression. Or that her hearing is not as good as it once was. But....

You see, I truly do understand what it feels like when a loved one is showing the signs of dementia. I didn't want to have those conversations either. But I had to. We (Mom and I) had to. I'm an only child, and so with that, I bear sole responsibility for her wellbeing.

So, we had the conversation. I know it was uncomfortable for Mom because it certainly was for me. She is aware that she's struggling, in fact, but unlike a lot of people who withdraw in an effort to hide it from everyone, she decided on her own, to be proactive about it; something for which I couldn't be prouder or more thankful.

She has been very proactive in terms of making financial arrangements, giving me her healthcare power of attorney, we even talked about potential future care needs. She lives in my home—in her own little apartment that is attached to us. That means for right now she is completely independent, she drives, she manages her own medication, and she manages her finances…and for the most part, she does a great job of it.

We did make a few adjustments, such as how much and for what purposes she uses her smart phone and computer. This was a bit uncomfortable for her to admit her need for supervision in this area, but it had to be done.

And during another conversation, before it got to the point where she asked me to promise I would never put her in a facility, I preempted it by saying, "Mom, please do not ask me to promise you that I will not, at some point, put you in a memory care facility."

"I hope to God, it never gets to that, but if it gets to the point where I cannot manage your needs at home, or you are a safety risk to herself, to me or my family, or if your needs could be better met in a facility where there are 24/7 caregivers who change shifts and they are fresh and not worn out, and they don't have other jobs, I will have to consider the possibility and might make the decision to do so."

Fortunately, and undoubtedly out of love for me, she said, "I hope it never gets to that point, but if it does, I understand." And to offer her some comfort, I reassured her that if it ever did get to that point. She wouldn't be aware of it, because the disease would be so advanced at that point, she wouldn't recognize me, or our home, or familiar surroundings.

I certainly never thought that this would be a conversation or a situation that I'd face, ten or twenty years ago. I really thought the only real health risks that ran in my family were colon cancer and heart disease. But as my aunts and uncles started to age, (my mom's the youngest of many children) more and more of her siblings were diagnosed with some form of dementia. The same thing happened on my dad's side. He is also the youngest of a large family. Many of his siblings have passed. Others are having cognitive issues, and some have been diagnosed with some type of dementia.

I know it's uncomfortable but have the conversation of what the future might look like. Know what your loved one's wishes are. I know that sounds grim and dreary, but not having the conversation doesn't make it go away. And quite truthfully, having the conversation is actually a bit freeing, because things that both of you are thinking about can be said. Getting it out there and talking it through provides some sense of relief. But again, remember that it's not going to be any easier if you wait. In fact, it probably will be more difficult.

If you have dementia in your family, I'm sure you can relate to what you've just read—that you've had these same thoughts, concerns, and questions. But that's why I'm here—why I wrote this book. I want you to know that you are not alone and that there is help and resources available for you and your loved one.

Dementia is an awful disease that destroys the mind, but it doesn't have to destroy your family.

Windows Perspective

Dad's dementia was nearing a point at which Mom was not going to be able to keep him home much longer. But after 65 years of marriage, raising four children, burying one daughter when she was just twenty-five years old and a new mom, and weathering the deaths of their parents, and a good number of other life events, she was bound and determined to postpone that day as long as possible. And by the grace of God and help from us kids, it was working. But then Mom got sick.

It started out as a cold, but quickly turned into a virus that settled in her heart. In less than a week she went from sniffling and coughing to clinging to life in the ICU 150 miles from home. Oh, and did I forget to mention this all took place in late April of 2020? Yep, we were faced with putting Dad in a care facility at home because we all still had to work, while monitoring Mom's condition from the parking lot of the hospital. Yes, the parking lot, because no one was allowed to visit—not even my sister who is a doctor in another hospital.

Mom died five days after being admitted to the hospital...alone.

And if that weren't bad enough, they wouldn't even allow us in the care facility to tell Dad. We had to literally stand outside his window and tell our dad, the man who had loved and cherished Mom all those years, but who could no longer feed or dress himself, that the love of his life was gone. The window! It was chilly, drizzling rain (very appropriate, don't you think), and just plain miserable.

In case you haven't already figured it out, the coronavirus has slammed the doors and windows of our lives shut in far too many ways. I know everyone has their own opinion on things, and that's fine. I totally respect that, but when we are reduced to window conversations like this, something is wrong. Terribly wrong.

My siblings and I decided then and there that we would do whatever it took to take care of Dad ourselves for whatever time he had left. Two days later, we took him to the cemetery to say goodbye to Mom, then took him home where he belonged. We had a schedule worked out that included some of the grown grandkids staying with him. But as it turned out, we didn't really need it. Sixteen days after we laid Mom to rest, we were sitting in the funeral home making Dad's final arrangements. The dementia and a broken heart took their toll. ~Steve

Because of COVID-19, I have found it necessary to facilitate a virtual support group that consists of people with family members currently residing in nursing homes—primarily because of dementia. Not unlike Steve and his family's experience, the nursing homes in this area have also resorted to 'window visits'.

Sometimes they encourage scheduled visits, but most of the time, spontaneous visits are okay, too, as long as all health precautions have been taken. It's hard and harsh, but because of the virus being so contagious, and because older people are among the most vulnerable, this is, according to the nursing home industry, the best they can do.

For some people, this 'window perspective' is enough. Their train of thought is that these window visits at least allow them to lay eyes on their loved one. They know that the window perspective will work better for their loved one than trying to 'force' something like SKYPE, ZOOM, Face Time, or Google Duo on them.

Think about it—if they are plagued with dementia, hearing loss, vision problems, arthritis, and/or other problems of the deteriorating body, how are they going to maneuver these apps…much less understand what they're doing?

The answer: They can't. More often than not, attempting something like this does more harm than good. For people with dementia, these platforms can be so disorienting and confusing, that some facilities have actually requested that families not attempt family visits like this.

Family members understand that, and in some cases, they (the family members) are as lost when it comes to trying to use these platforms as their loved one would be. Often times family members find it difficult to do window visits. Sometimes the visitors have their own mobility issues which make it difficult, or even impossible to do. Sometimes they feel that it puts an exclamation mark on what's going on, causing even more angst for their loved one.

In my practice as a neurology nurse practitioner, I started seeing the consequences of these window visits playing out in patients and their families—as you can imagine, these consequences were not good. That started me thinking about what I started calling the window perspective as something bigger than 'just' a way to visit your loved one in a pandemic-crazed world. I believe it symbolizes where you are you at in terms of dementia.

- Are you on the outside looking into a world you have no connection to? Like looking through the window of the nursing home you can't step foot inside of.

- Are you the caregiver of someone with mid to late-stage dementia? Looking through the window of their life knowing you are no longer a part of it-- from their perspective. You feel helpless and unable to do anything to change that.
- Are you looking through the window of dementia; see-sawing between facing the reality that you are starting down the road of dementia and denying this is actually happening to you? You feel isolated and alone—like you are looking through one of those windows that only goes one way.
- Are you on the outside of the window looking in at a disease that you know is real, but thankfully is not directly affecting your life in any way? Hoping it never does and distancing yourself from it in an effort to 'put curtains on that window'.

No matter what window you are looking through…what window perspective you have, chances are you are going to find your view changing at some point in your life. I use the term 'fluid situation' to describe this to my patients and their families. It is a fluid situation because it can change more than once. Over the course of your lifetime you may find yourself on the outside looking in, on the inside looking out, or even both…at the same time.

For example, when you leave the house each morning to go to work, you spend your day living a normal life that looks like the majority of the people around you. But when you go home and put on your 'caregiver hat', you feel anything but normal. You feel sad, isolated, restricted, confused, possibly frustrated, and most definitely tired.

But please know this: just like a house has many windows, you can, too. All of these windows are completely normal. Quite honestly, anyone who says that they don't experience these various emotions isn't being honest with themselves or anyone else.

The world of dementia, no matter which window you are looking through, is a painful, difficult world to live in. This fact is something I have said countless times to my support group members, to the family members of my patients, and to the patients themselves. And I will continue to say it until, well, forever. I want them to understand that it's okay to feel these things. They didn't choose to be a healthcare worker, yet as a caregiver, they are in the trenches, on the frontline, and are the eyes, and ears for the healthcare providers, i.e. doctors, nurses, and nurse practitioners like me.

As your loved one's caregiver or companion, we depend on you—your window perspective to tell us if something has changed. If something is wrong or 'off' with your loved one. If their normal is shifting. If their care plan needs to be adjusted or changed. Your window perspective helps us to see through the window more clearly. And in turn, it makes the patient's view from their window a little (or a lot) brighter. Even if only for a while.

My hope for you is that regardless of what window you are looking out of, that you're taking care of yourself, that you are making the connections you need to make, that you have an outlet for your questions, thoughts, and feelings, that you are not the only caregiver, and that you are being taken care of yourself—even if that means making deliberate choices to make it happen for yourself.

Remember: Dementia is something we need to take personally because it is personal.

Relocate

It was a rare day if I didn't spend at least a few hours with Granny. But if I didn't, you can be sure my phone or hers...or both rang once or twice

Yes, we were that tight. Peas in a pod is what she called us. When she started displaying signs of dementia (Alzheimer's), it was easy for my family and I to see because we were so invested in each other's lives. But for her kids (my aunts and uncles) and other grandkids who saw her once or twice a year, or who called now and again and on holidays, they couldn't (or wouldn't) see it.

In fact, before one of my cousins and his family, who hadn't seen her in over a year, came to visit for a couple of days, he called Granny and asked her to fix all his favorite foods while he was there!

In his defense, Granny was famous for her beyond-amazing cooking. Seriously, she was the best. But he was so out of touch with her, that he didn't know she'd not cooked anything beyond opening an occasional can of soup, for several months. She actually remembered the conversation and was fretting over it. She just 'wasn't up for all that' (her words).

I promptly called my cousin and politely (really) told him he and his wife needed to be prepared to do their own cooking when they came. He tried to tell me I was being over-protective, but I stood my ground and told him that putting that pressure on Granny was unfair...even cruel to Granny and that he needed to understand that visiting Granny was very different now.

He and his family came the following week and spent two nights. He said he could tell she was much frailer than she had been a year or two ago, but that he didn't think things were as bad as I made them out to be.

Whatever, I thought. I knew and my family and I were the ones taking the journey with her, so...so be it. ~Darla

The problem Darla's cousin had, is not uncommon when it comes to facing the reality of a loved one's dementia. I call it the need to relocate. Not literally, although if you need to change your physical location to help care for your loved one, then.... But that's a subject for another day, so let's stay on topic.

What I'm referring to is the need to meet your loved one where they are at instead of trying to keep them in the 'world' of yesterday or trying to transition them to fit into your world so you can care for them.

To further explain what I mean, let me share an example of something that happened to me recently. As I've already told you, my mom lives with me, and is having some undeniable problems with recall, finding her words, and following the right sequence of events. One challenge we frequently have is that she said she can't get into an account on her computer—the computer she really enjoys using. But because of her memory issues, it's common for her to not be able to access or get into a bank or an email account. But because she doesn't 'get' that the problem is her inability to complete the process properly, she tries to 'fix' the computer. She does things without me knowing and that she doesn't remember doing, so by the time I get involved, it's a hot mess.

When we first started having this problem on a (too) regular basis, I asked her what her password was. Being the organized woman that she is, she promptly pulled out a piece of paper on which she'd recorded her passwords. And people, I kid you not, she had 109 passwords written down. 1-0-9!!!!!!!!!!!! She had passwords for every site imaginable and she never used the same password twice. Now I agree that you should have a few different passwords depending on the level of sensitivity of the website, but 109?!?!? That's...that's...not good.

Lord have mercy, who could possibly remember all those passwords? For that matter, how many people do you know who could come up with that many passwords?

Apparently my mom could, because every time she signed up for something on a site asking for a password, she created one, and the rest, as they say, is history.

So, the first thing I did was clean everything up. Next we came up with a handful of passwords and wrote them down and listed the websites that went with each one underneath it.

And finally, I asked her... no, I begged her not to change anything.

The Mom of a few years ago would have complied with my request. The Mom who is experiencing a slow progressing dementia, however, does not. Or rather she cannot. It just isn't possible at this point.

She doesn't do it to be difficult. I know that, so between my daughter and I, we usually spend time every other week or so downstairs in her apartment retrieving passwords. In fact, that's what I did this morning before sitting down to write.

She was so frustrated, and honestly, so was I. Thankfully, though, I was able to keep my knee-jerk reaction in check and didn't say something like, "Are you serious?" Or "Not again!" No, this morning when I looked at her computer screen, my heart broke.

It broke because instead of multiple icons on the screen—shortcuts to all her favorite sites—there were four icons. Only four. I wanted to cry.

She's trying so hard to simplify her life so that she can actually hold on to her life, but it's not working, and I know it kills her to have to ask for help. I know it crushes her spirit to have to ask over and over and over again for help in getting the computer straightened out.

More than anything, though, I hope and pray we've never made her feel bad about it. So, I did what I always do. I took a deep breath, we talked about what she'd done, and then we retrieved the password...again.

This time it was different, though, because this time it dawned on me that we were missing the forest for the trees. We were trying to get her to stay in our world instead of us moving into hers.

I also realized that no matter how hard I try, I'll never be able to understand what she's going through. But that doesn't erase the fact that I need to accept and accommodate her condition. I need to move into her world so that I can make it a world that is safe, easy, and as stimulating as possible.

To help me do that, I took what is called a virtual dementia tour. A virtual dementia tour is your opportunity to experience what it's like to be disoriented, not recognizing textures, not being able to know what to do next, and several other things dementia patients live with on a 24/7 basis. And let me tell you, when you are done, you come out of that with a whole new appreciation, understanding, and compassion for your loved one. Be prepared, though, because it hurts. I started the tour with someone I knew. But because of some time overlap, she finished before I did. Completing the tour alone was awful. More realistic, but awful! I was lonely and terribly uncomfortable. I longed for something…anything familiar. You've probably noticed these same things with your loved one. For example, when you walk out of the room they become anxious; wanting to know where you are, even if you're only one room away. Sound familiar? Of course, it does.

As a caregiver your job…no, your privilege is to protect your loved one from feeling embarrassed and ashamed, and like an imposition. That is why I highly recommend a Virtual Dementia Tour. It can go a long way toward giving you the nudge and knowledge you need to relocate to their location so that life for everyone involved is a happier and healthier place to live. A win-win any way you look at it.

NOTE: Three virtual dementia tour sites worth checking out

https://www.nextavenue.org/take-virtual-dementia-tour/

https://www.oasissenioradvisors.com/senior-resources/virtual-dementia-tour/

https://www.secondwind.org/virtual-dementia-tourreg.html

Nutrition and Hydration

Snickers candy bars. Benny actually chose a Snickers bar over fried chicken, which had been his favorite food since he was a little boy. Chicken didn't even taste good anymore, he said with sadness in his voice. I think the first time he said that was when it really hit me that his dementia was real and that this was going to be our life now.

I'd seen it—the obsession with sweets—before. My sister in-law had done the same thing when she was alive. She couldn't get her fill of glazed donuts. I'd also seen the not-so-sweet side of dementia in my sister in-law's last couple of years. It was sad and it was hard—for her, for my brother, and for my niece and nephews and their families. For all of us who loved her.

I didn't let myself dwell on that part of it, though. Not because I was in denial. I just felt that it was better for both Benny and I to see the bright side of things—like eating candy bars without worrying about cavities, extra calories, or spoiling our dinner. He was 87 when his 'obsession' started, and I figured at that point he'd earned the right to eat whatever he wanted, whenever he wanted, and in whatever quantities he wanted. ~Betty

The topic of nutrition and hydration for dementia patients is a topic of major concern for their family members and caregivers. Their primary concern is that their loved one has an insatiable appetite for sweets. Regardless of whether or not they ever cared for sweets in the past, that's all they want now.

While there is definitely a lot we don't know about dementia, one thing we do know is that in addition to the changes in the brain (memory loss), there are also changes in the other parts of the body. One of those changes is the sensitivity of the taste buds. We also know that the ability to taste salty and sweet things lasts longer than the ability to taste sour, spicy, or bland foods. So, think about it—if you can't taste what you are eating, what's the point? Why go through the motions? Why not eat something you can taste and enjoy?

Eating habits aren't the only changes you'll see and experience in your loved one. These things don't happen overnight, or in the earliest stages of dementia. But as the disease progress there will be noticeable changes in their interests. What they once found interesting and enjoyable often becomes boring or frustrating. Sometimes they even become agitated when prodded to participate in these activities.

So, what are you supposed to do about their obsession with sweets? Ignore it? Feed into it (pun intended)? Battle it like you did with your kids when they were toddlers? And do the benefits of insisting on a healthy diet outweigh the benefits of allowing them this form of independence— retaining their right to choose?

I don't mean to muddy the waters, but there really is no single correct answer. As I said in the first chapter, we know we can't stop the progression of dementia, nor can we reverse it. The best we can do is manage the disease in such a way that the journey will be as comfortable as possible for someone suffering from this awful, awful disease. That means as caregivers, we have to find the balance that works best. Or as parenting experts say when dealing with kids, we have to learn to choose our battles and the 'weapons' with which we 'fight'.

The first weapon I suggest pulling out of your arsenal is negotiation. "After you eat 'this' you can have two of 'those'." Negotiation is a good way to 'sneak' in some nutrient-rich calories, but it is also an essential if your loved one is battling another common disease among the elderly—diabetes.

Diabetes is a disease affecting blood sugar (glucose). Blood pressure, weight, and physical activity, as well as diet, are contributing factors for the onset of this disease. Dietary restrictions, as in low sugar intake, are essential for keeping glucose levels in the 'safe zone'.

Negotiating food choices is also important because wise food choices (avoiding carb overload) reduces what we commonly call brain fog when carbs and sugars are our primary source of calories. Surely you can understand the importance of this in someone who is already having cognitive issues. Following the brain fog is fatigue, brought on by the drop in sugar levels. Then when they pop more sweets, it starts all over again. The constant rising and falling of sugar levels works against them by intensifying mood instability and disorientation. The instant gratification of satisfying their sweet tooth ends up making matters worse in every other way.

The solution is easy. Focus on protein. We're going to assume that your loved one doesn't have kidney disease, a heart condition, bowel issues, or some other pre-existing health condition that requires them to eat a diet lower in protein that the average person should eat. So, if your loved one is required to limit protein per doctor's orders, do NOT make these changes. Follow doctor's orders.

If, however, that is not the case, you will find that upping their protein intake balances out their intake of sweets by working to keep blood sugar levels stable and consistent instead of letting it spike and crash from the high carb and sugar intake.

Great, you say. You're all for it. You know what needs to be done but convincing your candy-eater is another story. You know what to do—it's how to do it that has you stymied.

My suggestion in dealing with this problem, is to manage through moderation and trial and error. Don't deny them their sweets. But offer other fun foods (foods with different textures, bright colors, and easy for them to feed themselves.

NOTE: There's a list of suggestions at the end of this chapter to help you get started in thinking along these lines.

Additional suggestions for managing their intake of sweets include:

- Limit the portion size. You can even do this without their realizing it. A one-cup container with one big scoop looks like a lot more ice cream than a bigger cereal bowl with two scoops.
- Instead of sugary snacks, give them fruit once or twice a day.
- Make homemade sweet treats instead of giving them store-bought versions. For example, homemade peanut butter cookies with miniature

chocolate chips are much healthier than chocolate/peanut butter cups.

- Use honey instead of refined sugar to sweeten things.
- Cut the amount of sugar in a recipe in half. *Pinterest or cookbooks for diabetics will give you some great ideas on how to do this without sacrificing taste.
- DON'T use artificial sweeteners. These are nothing more than chemicals that provide a small level of instant gratification but cause the body to crave sweets.
- Try nutritional drinks; you're going to get a lot of dense calories in a small amount of liquid. Ensure is really good, or Glucerna if you're diabetic. CAUTION: Too many nutritional drinks can cause some GI issues.
- Dried fruit. It's higher in sugar, so again, you'll need to put some limitations in place, but it's better than refined sugar.
- Nuts (if they can digest them) toasted with a bit of honey or sugar/cinnamon will satisfy their sweet tooth and give them the protein boost they need.

This isn't always going to be easy, but you have to be patiently firm, because they have to eat. Calories are important.

Calories translate into energy. So, while balanced meals are definitely your goal, if they refuse to eat the stuff that is good for them, you are going to have to let them eat the food that tastes good to them. Otherwise, they will become lethargic, experience an even greater lag in energy, and become even more despondent and confused than they already are.

Now let's move on to the subject of hydration...

Hydration is even more important than sound nutrition. Without proper hydration nothing's going to work properly. And by hydration, I mean water. Water is an interesting beverage—you either love it or you don't. If your loved one doesn't like water, you are going to have to come up with some way to make sure they drink plenty of it, anyway.

- Infuse it with fruits, berries, or vegetables.
- Add a splash of orange, lemon, or lime juice to give it an added bit of zing (taste).
- Hot water with honey and/or lemon hydrates and helps with bowel function.

NOTE: Pre-packaged flavored water contains chemicals. Don't do it. OR, if you think it will help, cut regular water with a bit of this flavored water.

NOTE: Don't do carbonated water.

Say it with me: Hydration is essential. With hydration, however, comes another problem: bladder control issues. The issue of bladder control (incontinence) is a common problem among people with dementia for two reasons:

- Loss of memory causes them to forget they shouldn't wet themselves
- Loss of muscle tone in the bladder makes it difficult for them to 'hold it' long enough to get to the bathroom. Diminished mobility only adds to this problem.

Water is important because it flushes the toxins from your system—toxins that cause confusion in anyone, regardless of their age or medical condition. Water is also the key ingredient to clearing your kidneys and all the waste that is caused by everyday activities and your body's metabolism.

People often ask me how they can tell if they or their loved one is getting enough water. The easiest way to tell is to 'tent' your skin. This is done by pinching the skin on the top of your hand while it is lying flat on a table.

Pinch the skin in the middle; gently pulling it upward to make a 'tent'. Release it. If it falls back into place without hesitation, you (or your loved one) is fine. If it stays up, or is slow to fall back into place, you (or your loved one) need to up your water intake.

Another way to tell is the color of their urine. First thing in the morning our urine is naturally darker yellow. By early afternoon it should be clear or almost clear in color. If it's not, the closer it is to the color it was first thing in the morning, the more you need to increase your (or your loved one's) water intake. Note: some medications and vitamins can cause your urine to appear a hint of yellow so be mindful of this when evaluating hydration status.

I want to stress here, that water is the only thing that counts when working toward proper hydration. Tea, coffee, juice, or soda do not. There are several great reasons to drink tea, and a cup or two of coffee in the morning is also good for promoting bowel movements, stimulates the nervous system, benefits liver function, and a few other things, as well. Juice and soda, on the other hand, are empty (nutritionally void) calories that add unwanted and unneeded sugars and chemicals to the body. I'm not saying they should never have these things but keep them to a minimum.

NOTE: The exception is pure juices (no sugar added).

Water is the only beverage that prevents urinary tract and kidney infections. Of course you know these infections are unpleasant, uncomfortable, and can lead to more serious, even fatal health condition. But what you may not know is that urinary tract and kidney infections cause confusion, disorientation, and possibly even hallucinations.

My uncle is the 'poster child' for this situation. He has dementia and lives in a nursing home because he requires a level of care that is beyond what our family is able to provide at home. He got a urinary tract infection that went undetected for several days, despite presenting some common symptoms including a low-grade fever.

By the time he was taken to the hospital the urinary tract infection was a full-blown kidney infection that traveled to his bloodstream. This is what is referred to as being 'septic'. Sepsis (being septic) damaged his heart (a common occurrence with sepsis) and he has now been diagnosed with heart failure.

As I write this, we don't know how this is going to turn out. But what we do know is that it won't be good. It is highly possible he won't survive. If he does, the best we can hope for is a new normal. But because an infection of any kind causes cognitive decline, his new normal (and the family's) will be a much lower baseline of cognitive memory and capabilities.

A few side notes on this matter:

- Two-thirds of all dementia patients in the country are women, which is most likely due to the fact that women tend to live longer than men, and dementia is primarily an age-related disease.
- Women have a significantly greater problem with weak bladder muscles.

This means that increasing water intake also increases the frequency of urination. In turn, the added frequency to 'go' will probably cause more incontinence problems. Yes, this is going to cause more work for you and other caregivers. And yes, it is likely to cause those in the early to mid-stages of dementia added embarrassment, but it's something you'll have to work through, because ultimately, hydration is of the utmost importance.

To 'work through' the situation includes the option of disposable adult briefs. If your loved one is resistant to, or refuses this option, regular bathroom breaks at specific times after drinking, water-resistant pads in their chair and bed, and patience…lots of patience are about all that's left. But hey, we do what we have to do, right? This is one of those 'relocation' issues we've already discussed.

None of us wants that for our loved ones. And since it is one of the few things we can actively control (and avoid) by making sure our loved one stays hydrated, all I can say is why wouldn't you do that. Why wouldn't you try to make sure your loved one gets the water intake they need?

Creative Foods List:

- Chocolate covered raisins and nuts

- Cheese cubes (you might want to consider getting the ones shaped like Mickey Mouse)
- Lunchables, because they are easy to handle, but be mindful of the high sodium content in some of them
- Egg, cheese, and bacon muffins (mix the ingredients and pour into muffin tins and bake)
- Fruit pizza
- Oatmeal with chocolate chips
- Homemade cookies using healthier ingredients (applesauce, honey)
- Meatballs
- Pudding
- Peanut butter and crackers
- Deviled eggs
- Yogurt (no sugar) with fresh fruit

To Know or not to Know…That is the Question

"What you don't know won't hurt you, but what you do know can." This old adage is one of those things that rings true no matter how you look at it. But when it comes to knowing if you are pre-dispositioned to Alzheimer's or any other disease, I definitely think you are better off not knowing. I know everyone doesn't feel that way, but I'm basing my opinion on experience.

My aunt had Huntington's disease. Huntington's is a type of dementia that robs you of your memory, your ability to see things from a logical and reasonable point of view, and it shoves you into a dark hole of depression.

My aunt, a woman with the gentlest, kindest, heart, and who loved and adored her family, became so despondent that she took her own life. It was devastating to all of us, but her kids were feeling a lot more than grief. They were also scared. What if they had Huntington's? Like their mom, their maternal grandpa, and their maternal great grandma?

Both boys decided against testing.

One of the girls was tested several years ago, the other one less than a year ago. Both girls have the gene.

One reacted by spending about a year trying to outwit Huntington's by overeating, smoking, and doing the 'couch potato' routine.

She decided to make sure something else took her down before Huntington's did. After about a year, though, she realized how dangerous and ridiculous that was, so she started being proactive instead of foolishly reactive.

The other daughter responded by taking a proactive approach from the get-go.

Both girls say they wish they didn't know—that they would have been vigilant (not paranoid) about watching for early signs and symptoms, but that they didn't 'know' it was a near-certainty that at some point they will become their mom.

Their experience reinforced what I already knew about myself—that knowing something like that will turn me into a paranoid mess. I would be so worried about what possibly lies ahead that I would miss the here and now.
~Lisa

Should you, or should you not consider having genetic testing to discern the probability of developing Alzheimer's disease?

That's what most people would call a 'loaded question'. At best, it's controversial, but it is also something I believe people need to discuss. Not necessarily whether or not to be tested, but rather their feelings on the subject, what they would do with the information, and so forth.

Before we go any farther, I want you to now understand that the following information is strictly my opinion. My opinion is based on my knowledge in the medical field, AND on my own personal thoughts and feelings.

Keeping that in mind, I want you to use the following information in a way that will best serve you and your family.

Looking at Alzheimer's from a scientific perspective

Let's start by making sure you understand the most basic facts about Alzheimer's disease not 'just' generalized dementia, because that's where I'm going to focus my attention.

I'm going to give you an elementary level lesson in the science of genetics as it pertains to Alzheimer's.

For starters, let's break the disease down into two parts— early-onset, which means that the symptoms develop before age 65, and late-onset, which develops after age 65. Then within each of those, you need to remember that there are different stages of Alzheimer's. Early stage is the presentation of the beginning signs and the stage at which the patient has more periods of lucidity than not. Eventually the disease progresses (if you want to call it that), to late-stage Alzheimer's. Late-stage patients have little or no memory and have lost all (or nearly all) ability to care for themselves.

APOE

APOE is the 'name' given to genes we all have. We get one APOE gene from each parent to form the APOE chromosome. APOE gene produces a protein that is essential for healthy brain function. But not all APOE genes are alike. The medical world has assigned them numbers, i.e. APOE 2, 3, and 4.

We don't know why APOE 4 increases a person's likelihood of developing Alzheimer's disease, but the proof is irrefutable that it does. What's more, people who inherit APOE 4 from one parent, but not the other, are less likely than those who inherit APOE 4 from both parents.

Age increases probability

Countless unsolved mysteries and unanswered questions about Alzheimer's plague medical researchers and doctors. One thing, however, is for sure and for certain: The older you get, the greater your chances are of developing Alzheimer's. That's the way it is. Age is not in our favor when talking about Alzheimer's and other dementia-related diseases. So, while getting old isn't a guarantee to falling victim to Alzheimer's, we can safely say that the aging, i.e. deteriorating body has something to do with its ability to attack and destroy.

PSEN1 and PSEN2

PSEN1, and PSEN2 are genes that control the manufacturing of another protein in the brain that works alongside the protein controlled by the APOE genes. APOE genes are linked with late-onset Alzheimer's. PSEN genes are linked with early-onset Alzheimer's.

In the case of PSEN1 and PSEN2, if you inherit either of these genes from just one parent, you have a near 100% chance of developing early-onset Alzheimer's.

News like that is unsettling and upsetting. Frightening, even. But it can also be helpful when it comes to both business and personal decisions. I say this because knowing that you are all but certain of developing early-onset (before age 65) Alzheimer's gives you the opportunity, i.e. the push you need, to get your business and personal affairs in order while YOU still have the wherewithal and abilities to make and execute those decisions according to YOUR wishes and expectations.

Other genes

The APOE and PSEN genes are just two genes that are under close scientific study and scrutiny in terms of Alzheimer's research.

There are other genes being studied in an effort to find out as much as possible about other forms of dementia, because remember, Alzheimer's is a type of dementia, but not the only one.

Summing it all up

Up to now, the content of this chapter has been factual based on research and studies that have been proven to be accurate and correct. Now it's time for me to insert my opinion on what you should do with this information.

Remember: my opinion, though based on experience and professional knowledge, is still just my opinion. You are the only one who can decide what is right for you.

My opinion is actually two-fold, depending on:

- What type of Alzheimer's you are wanting to be tested for
- Your reasons for being tested

#1: If you have reason to believe, or are justifiable concerned about early-onset (before age 65) Alzheimer's, Huntington's, or some other inherited form of dementia that often strike people prior to their 'golden years', then I suggest getting tested.

Like I said earlier, knowing what your chances of developing dementia during a period in life when you are making personal, business, financial, and relational decisions and are living an active, mobile life, can be extremely helpful. Not only will you have the confidence that you are making your own choices and decisions about the way things are done now and in the possibly-not-so-bright future.

Knowing what your chances of facing dementia will also allow you to prepare in advance for your care. You can make adjustments and renovations to your home to allow you to age in place, you can liquidate assets so that they are not swallowed up by the expenses of your healthcare, and you can prepare your family for what might be coming.

Last but not least, you can take decisive and deliberate actions NOW to ward off dementia:

- Eat a healthy diet and stay hydrated
- Exercise
- Keep your mind sharp by being social (conversations), working puzzles of all kinds, reading, playing trivia games, and engaging in hobbies and work or volunteer activities
- Don't smoke and keep alcohol to a minimum
- Take care of your body in an effort to ward off diabetes, vascular disease, and other conditions that tend to increase one's chances of developing dementia

#2: If you are more concerned about late-onset Alzheimer's or other types of dementia that tend to strike later in life, don't do the testing. Instead, spend your time focusing on enjoying life and making the most of it, vs. stressing, worrying, and 'what-iffing' yourself into a state of anxiety or depression. Or as a wise old woman I once knew said,

"Why go borrowing trouble, when there's plenty to be had for free?"

More often than not, people who get tested for late-onset dementia end up causing themselves more harm (angst) than good. Every time they forget the littlest thing—whether an item on their shopping list, or their great-grandbaby's birthday—they are plagued with doubt. Was this lapse in memory just part of getting older or due to being distracted?

Or is it almost here—is Alzheimer's setting in?

Now ask yourself, "Do I really want to live like that?"

No one does.

That is why my humble advice to you is to think long and hard about both sides of this fence before approaching the gate. Once you know, you can't unknow. But if you don't know, you can live wisely, pay attention to your body, and fill your heart with joy and great memories of each and every day you are given. So, like the song says…

"Don't worry. Be happy."

FYI: There are companies such as 23andMe and Ancestry.com (along with several others) that offer genetic testing for a wide variety of diseases, including Alzheimer's.

CBD and Dementia

Dementia is an awful disease. It's the worst, if you ask me, and I know. I've lived it with my grandma, my dad, my father in-law, two aunts, my grandma in-law, and have had several friends over the years who have slipped in a world in which none of us is really a part of. I hate it. I can't imagine how scary it is for that person when they are at the stage when they know something's not right but can't quite put their finger on it. Even worse, they can't keep it from happening, no matter how hard they try. And then there's the rest of us—those of us who love these people and try desperately to help them hold on to reality. But we don't have any more power to stop the progression than they do.

I know science is trying to find a way to help dementia patients, but so far, they've not come up with any long-term solutions or better yet, a cure. I think that's why so many people are willing to try just about anything to keep dementia from taking over for as long as possible. Holistic treatments, alternative medicine like herbs, eating a lot of certain foods, strict vitamin regimens, and now even CBD. People's opinions about CBD are all over the map, but when you are losing your grip on reality or watching a loved one lose theirs, you aren't nearly as concerned with propriety or traditional treatments as you used to be.

That's where Annette was 'at'. She had given the doctors every opportunity, she said, to find an approved drug to help slow her husband's dementia down. These drugs have been successful in other cases, but he had an allergic reaction to the two they tried, so she decided to take matters into her own hands and try CBD. It's only been a couple of weeks, so the jury is still out, but from what I've read, I think it's definitely worth a try. ~Ron

These days you see CBD advertisements everywhere you look. It is supposedly the miracle for whatever ails you. Arthritis? Mood swings? Problems sleeping? Dementia? Proponents of CBD claim to have the answer for it all.

Before we get into the possibility (or not) of CBD's effectiveness in dealing with dementia, lets' take a few minutes to make sure we know what CBD is and is not. But before we do that, I want to make a little disclaimer here and say that I am not an expert on the matter, nor am I endorsing or warning you against the use of CBD. I'm just giving you some factual scientific information.

What is cannabis

CBD comes from the plant called cannabis. When people think of cannabis, they automatically think about the part of the plant that produces THC, the psychoactive component of cannabis. That has been proven to do a great deal of harm to the body. Harm as in…

- Damage blood cells
- Increase the risk of some cancers
- Diminish short-term memory
- Hinder creativity
- Cause hallucinations
- Damage brain cells

*According to "Men's Journal" "The Street.com"

THC also gives you a 'high' that increases your appetite, aka, gives you the munchies. But there's another part of the cannabis plant, that when genetically modified, the plant, does not have these same negative effects.

I will be the first to admit I don't understand all the technical aspects of it. But simply put, they take the THC out of the plant and then extract the desired CBD in the form of an oil. The oil is then used to make edibles, tinctures, or leave it in oil form. And according to the cannabis experts, this is non-psychoactive.

The experts say that the level of THC is no more than 0.3%. But even at that, you need to be aware that if you use it and are subjected to a drug screening, the trace amounts (which probably fluctuates depending on who and how the products are made and who makes them), may still cause you to test positive.

We have receptors for cannabis

What's interesting or even strange (to me, anyway) is that we have receptors in our body that are able to interact with the chemicals in cannabis—the non-hallucinatory elements—in a non-harmful way. Or so it appears in some cases, anyway.

The receptors are CB1 and CB2 and each one has its own agenda. The CB1 receptor is found primarily in the central nervous system—your brain, spinal cord, and your nerves. CB2 is mostly found in your GI tract but is also present in your brainstem and your hippocampus. FYI, the hippocampus is the part of the brain that converts short term memory to long term memory.

As for how these receptors respond to CBD, working with the receptors, it has been shown to decrease brain inflammation, decrease oxygen build-up, and work like an antioxidant, which ultimately improves brain stimulation. Not like a stimulant, though.

Another 'not' in this equation is 'not approved'…yet. You need to know that the FDA (Food and Drug Administration) has not yet approved the use of CBD for Alzheimer's disease or any other types of dementia. I feel I need to tell you, though, that more often than not, when you read people's testimonies about using the non-THC enriched cannabis in the early stages of Alzheimer's, they report an improvement in their mood, experience less anxiety, seem to be less forgetful, and sleep more soundly.

Each of these things is beneficial to everyone. But for someone with dementia, getting regular and sound sleep is extremely important. Better rest usually translates into being more cooperative, not as easily agitated, and better able to comprehend and carry out simple instructions (early and mid-stages).

The benefits sound appealing, but many (if not most) people are still against using CBD because of the fear of becoming addicted or experiencing other harmful side effects that outweigh the benefits they might derive from it. And then there's that issue of it not being approved by the FDA, or readily available in most areas of the country.

The only answer I have for you on that is that the type of CBD we're talking about his is non-addictive and from a medical standpoint there is no dependency created by using it. From all I've been able to gather, the best forms tend to be the oils. However, you need to know that unlike a pain pill that gives you relief 20 or 30 minutes after you take it, the benefits of CBD are not as instantaneous.

Reports show that it seems to take several weeks before the CBD oil has any therapeutic effect. It has to accumulate in your system for three to four weeks of daily use before there are any noticeable benefits.

CBD is a drug so, as is the case with all types of medications whether prescribed or purchased over the counter, you need to be aware of any possible drug interactions with everything you are taking. If for no other reason, I cannot emphasize enough how important it is to discuss taking CBD with your healthcare provider and or your pharmacist because the last thing you want is to have a negative and possibly toxic reaction to mixing CBD with your prescribed medications.

Let me repeat that…it is particularly important that you have a conversation with whoever is managing your health before adding anything to your regimen—CBD or anything else. Other things to keep in mind about taking CBD:

- As long as it is not THC-enriched, you do not need a prescription for CBD.
- You can find CBD anywhere—including your local gas station/convenience store and online, but that doesn't mean it's all the same…or safe.
- You get what you pay for. CBD is not inexpensive. You can typically plan to spend about $60 per month to get quality CBD.
- Just like anything else, quality is key. If there is a lot of sediment in the CBD oil, the quality is poor.
- Be aware of and adherent to any and all laws concerning the use and possession of any forms of CBD in your state.

The long and short of it all

I'm not saying I think CBD is a bad idea. I'm not saying I think CBD is a good idea. I'm not saying the claims that say CBD is a 'wonder drug' are true or false…exaggerated or accurate. I can't really do that because I don't know. But what I am saying is that sometimes we need to think outside the box. Sometimes we need to challenge the thinking of conventional medicine. After all, there was a time when people thought antibiotics were witches brew and leeches were the only way to purify the blood.

On the other hand, we need to remember that the FDA hasn't approved it…yet. So, maybe conventional medicine is the best option for you. At least for now—until we have more information.

So, what do you think?

Have I been able to clear up any misinformation or questions you had about CBD and its use for dementia? Or have I just muddied the waters more than they already were? I hope I've been able to help, at least in some small way. At the very least, if you've been thinking about CBD as an alternative medication, I hope I've given you the nudge you need to do some thorough research and to discuss the possibility with your healthcare professionals.

Hallucinations Happen

I will never forget the look of confusion in Grandma Mary's eyes, or the sound of desperation in her voice as she told me about seeing Grandpa Doyle and two other dear friends—all of whom had been dead for over twenty years.

"They were here," she said. "We talked, I had some cake, and played a few rounds of dominos," she said. Then pausing and taking a deep breath and letting it out, she said, "But they weren't, were they?"

I didn't say anything. I didn't have to because she answered her own question. "I know they weren't. I know they're dead. But when they are here, it's so real. I can smell the aftershave, and Maudie's perfume she always wore. I can feel Doyle's hand squeeze mine the way he always did when he thanked me for a meal or dessert. And then once they leave, it takes a while to decide whether or not it really happened. It's the strangest thing I've ever experienced. And scary."

Grandma Mary's hallucinations only got worse. She even left one day in her car to take them on a Sunday drive. She got lost and drove around for what we later determined to be about two hours.

She finally 'snapped out of it', recognized a familiar landmark, and drove home. She called us that evening and told Wayne (my husband/her grandson) to come get the keys to her car. She was never going to drive it again.
~Dana

I think the term hallucinations tends to conger up frightening thoughts in people who aren't having them. Somewhat surprisingly, though, most people are like Grandma Mary whom you just 'met'.

They are not frightened by their hallucinations. In fact, I've actually had a handful of patients tell me they don't want their hallucinations to away. They find them somewhat comforting.

Going back to Grandma Mary, you can see how that might be true. In the moment, being able to enjoy time with her beloved husband and friends felt good.

Older people are often very lonely because their spouse, as well as many (if not most) of their friends (peers who are their age) die, leaving them feeling like an antique on a shelf. So to have a few brief periods of joy from 'spending time with them', is nothing to be scared of in the least.

Not so with us—those who are on the outside looking in. Knowing our loved one is hallucinating can't help but make us anxious and sad, because we know something's wrong. In turn, that causes our knee-jerk reaction to want to make the hallucinations stop so that our loved one won't be 'broken'.

Trust me, I get that.

But when my patients tell me they are experiencing hallucinations, one of the first questions I ask is, "Are they frightening?" If they aren't, we don't treat them. And here's why….

ONE: The medications used to treat hallucinations are not necessarily benign. They are antipsychotic, aka, neuroleptic drugs. They come with their own set of issues (side effects) that are often worse than the hallucinations themselves.

They carry something called a Black Box Warning. A Black Box Warning is something that the FDA (Food and Drug Administration) applies to a medication or device that is the most stringent type of alert they can issue. Its purpose is to inform the public and healthcare industry about potential side-effect, such as injury or death.

The Black Box Warning associated with this class of drugs is that it is not indicated for dementia-related psychosis, which includes hallucinations in persons 65 years of age or older

See the problem? That is why I tell people it's about choice; weighing the risks and benefits, because ultimately, aside from the obvious concern of safety, it is about quality of life. If your loved one is agitated, or hallucinating, and these hallucinations are frightening, then medication would enhance the quality of their life. But if they aren't causing negative behaviors, then why risk it?

Another fact you need to be aware of is that some forms of dementia are actually characterized by hallucinations. For example, Lewy body dementia, or Parkinson's related dementia, or even vascular dementia all cause hallucinations on a somewhat regular basis.

With Alzheimer's disease, we know that in the moderate and advanced stages, hallucinations are also quite common, but you don't typically see hallucinations in the early stages.

TWO: Hallucinations can also be an indicator of infection. If, however, you treat the hallucinations because you think they are solely dementia-related, you might actually be putting your loved one at risk for serious complications due to an untreated infection. Possibly even death.

If your loved one hasn't been talking about hallucinations or given you any indication that they are hallucinating, but suddenly start to do so, the first thing I would recommend is to get them evaluated for infection—usually a urinary tract infection.

I know that sounds extreme, but it's not. It is actually quite common. As we get older, we lose some of the signs we have when we're younger warning us of a urinary tract infection: distinct lower abdominal cramping or burning with urination.

Sometimes in dementia patients, those symptoms may still present themselves, but the patient doesn't think about why they don't feel good or remember to tell someone. It is also not uncommon to have absolutely no symptoms of infection except acute confusion and even possible hallucinations.

So remember, if your loved one doesn't typically hallucinate, but suddenly begins to do so, don't waste any time in taking them to be evaluated.

FYI: Unless they spike a temperature, a trip to the ER isn't necessary. A call to their primary care physician to report the symptoms will usually suffice. They will collect a urine sample, and if infection is present, prescribe antibiotics. Once the antibiotics are in their system for a few days, the infection will typically subside, as will the hallucinations.

Delusion and hallucination…the two words are not interchangeable

The general public, which most likely includes you, is often guilty of interchanging the words 'hallucination' with 'delusion'. It's a bit like misusing 'there' and 'their'...and 'they're'...but with a LOT more at stake.

A hallucination is seeing or hearing something that isn't there for a brief period of time. And then it is gone. A delusion is typically a sense of paranoia—a belief that something is true, which in reality, is not. A delusion isn't something they just see or hear, but rather it is something they think or believe. And in turn, those thoughts and beliefs cause them to think they see or hear things that aren't really there.

Here are a couple of examples to help you distinguish between the two:

Hallucination: A dementia patient who sees and talks to her brother who was killed overseas in Viet Nam, or who says he hears his dog barking and calls for him...even though the dog died several years prior.

Delusion: A person who is convinced that the people in the care facility are aliens trying to abduct him/her and take them to another planet, or that the nurse assigned to their care is really the daughter she gave up for adoption as a teenager.

If your loved one starts becoming paranoid or having delusions they need to be evaluated immediately. Sometimes delusions are also caused by infection.

The most common reason for delusional thoughts in dementia patients, though is adverse interactions between their medications. This is completely treatable and fixable, so don't delay in putting off a trip to the doctor for an evaluation and consultation/review of their medications. Delusional thoughts are hard to deal with. Unlike hallucinations which tend to be good thoughts, (most of the time, anyway), delusions are scary and cause anxiety and fear.

FYI: Antipsychotics or neuroleptics such as Risperdal, or Seroquel, Geodon, Haldol, and Abilify have been known to cause patients to become delusional.

*This statement is NOT meant to be taken as medical advice and should not take the place of talking to your doctor about your medications and the possible interactions between them. This statement is NOT meant to encourage a patient from stopping a medication. Always consult your healthcare provider before starting or stopping any medication (prescribed or otherwise).

As is the case with medications for hallucinations, it's all about weighing the risks against the benefits and vice versa. Medications for these conditions can be helpful and provide much-needed relief. Each patient's situation and needs must be looked at carefully and specifically to determine what is best for them.

To sum it all up

When it comes to deciding whether or not your loved one should take medication for hallucinations, talk to them if at all possible. Help them think out loud to determine whether or not the hallucinations they have are:

- Causing them to have more trouble distinguishing between what is real and what isn't
- Putting themselves or anyone else at risk for harm

- Causing them to be anxious, sad, depressed, irritable, or agitated
- Diminishing the quality of their life
- Making it difficult for them to age in place (stay in their own home or current living situation)

Or...

- Giving them a bit of respite from the realities of growing old 'alone'
- Giving them some peace of mind or comfort about life after death
- Not causing any additional angst or depression

Based on the answers to those questions you should be able to make the best decision for your loved one. I also know that as a caregiver or a concerned and involved family member, you will find that saying something like, "Tell them it's time to go because "You need your rest", or even something more direct such as, "They aren't really there, but it's nice to pretend once in a while, isn't it." goes a long way toward making sure your loved one isn't unnecessarily medicated, while at the same time, allowing them to feel respected and maintain their dignity.

What's So Funny

One morning I went in to finish helping Granny get dressed for the day. I'd already laid out her clothes but needed to get her clean underwear out of the dryer. As I came out of the laundry room, Granny was walking out of her bedroom...without a stitch of clothing on! "Granny! What are you doing?" I asked.

My extremely modest Granny looked at herself, realized what she was doing, and...laughed. It wasn't just a chuckle or a snicker. She laughed. Then after a few seconds, she said, "I guess I forgot to put my clothes on," she said, then turned around and followed me back to the bedroom and let me get her dressed. ~Darla

Have you noticed that sometimes older people tend to laugh at inappropriate times? Or at things that aren't really all that funny? Sometimes they laugh in place of giving an answer. If you've not experienced that, you probably think I'm the one with memory problems, but I'm not. This really is a 'thing', but despite my best efforts and a lot of searching for answers, I cannot tell you for sure why it's a 'thing'. Instead, I'll tell you why I think it is.

I think older people insert laughter in place of an answer to fill space.

I've seen it happen time and again with my mother. When I ask her a question, she often laughs, even though the answer she needs to give doesn't pair well with laughter. I think she's laughing in order to:

- Give herself time to remember the right answer.

- Give herself time to think of something to say besides, "I don't know".
- Deal with the fact that once more she's been defeated by her loss of memory; softening the blow by trying to make light of it.
- Make herself feel less sad over what used to be but is no more, aka, her sharp mind.

If that's the case, then perhaps putting some laughter in place of an answer, or inserting it before they answer, makes them feel a bit more normal.

In addition to the laughter, I've also noticed that many of my patients talk around something.

What I mean by that is when I ask a question that they don't know the answer to, they avoid answering by talking about something they do know. This is referred to as tangential speech.

Example:

Me: "Can you tell me who our current President is?"

Patient: "I still remember how aggravated I got when Walter Cronkite interrupted "As the World Turns" that day President Kennedy was shot and killed. But as soon as I saw the look on his face I knew something bad had happened and I decided the Hughes family could wait."

Do you see what happened? Not only did she get out of answering my question (which she probably didn't know the answer to), she completely changed the subject to something she could talk about—and was more interesting, to boot!

After mulling these observations over in my mind for a while, I decided that instead of just observing and categorizing these fillers as 'just something that happens with age', we need to do something about them…for the good of our loved one.

By now you know me well enough to know that I'm not going to just leave you hanging with that statement. No way! Now I'm going to tell you what I think we should do when it happens. Or in some cases, before it happens.

DISCLAIMER: I cannot take full credit for the following ideas and information. A lot of what I'm going to share with you is my 'translation' of a video by Diana Waugh titled, "How to Talk to Someone with Dementia". It's a bit lengthy (almost an hour), but I strongly encourage people to watch it, because she has some pertinent and wise things to say. https://www.youtube.com/watch?v=ilickabmjww

One: I think we should look at the questions we are asking and consider asking them differently. Instead of asking someone with dementia fact-based questions, ask them to tell you how they feel about something. Most of the time you'll get enough information from their answer to give you the facts you need. Or if not, you can try to guide the conversation in that direction without making them feel inadequate.

Two: Don't start with short-term memory questions. When we do that, we're setting them up for failure. Shame on us. And by 'us', I mean, me, too. Short-term memory is the first thing to go, so why would we expect them to be able to do that? Think about it—my patient didn't know who the president is—the one she saw on the news less than an hour earlier, but she knew JFK's name, the details of his death, and the names of the people on the soap opera she was watching that day!!! That's short-term vs. long-term.

Three: The goal of our conversations with our loved one should be to validate them. To make them feel that they still have worthwhile contributions to make to our lives. To keep them engaged vs. letting them retreat into their own little world. To empower them. To help them stay sharp and focused. To extend the quality of their life. Am I right? Of course, I am!

But when we ask all the wrong questions, or ask the right questions the wrong way, we are defeating the purpose for asking them in the first place. All of the things we don't want them to feel, we cause them to feel.

Try this

Diana's video, as well as some other research I've done, has given me some incredibly useful tips on how to have enjoyable conversations with my mom and my patients. Here are a couple I found especially helpful:

ONE: Say, "I was thinking about the time we (fill in the blank)." This gives your loved one the springboard to recall the incident without the pressure of feeling like they have to...or have to get it exactly right. Even a simple "Yes," or "That's nice" is a lot more dignified for them than to have to say "No" when you just say, "Do you remember..."

TWO: Choose your time wisely. Recognize when your loved one is at their daily peak in terms of clarity and cognitive function. For some, it's right after breakfast, for others it is mid to late afternoon.

Studies have been done on why this is, but that's a topic for another day. The point I want to make here is to save the important stuff for when they are most alert. The rest of the time can be spent talking about things they can recall from long-term memory, looking at old pictures, or playing games that will keep them talking...and laughing.

We've come full circle back to using laughter as a filler. Use it as a cue—especially if the possibility of your loved one's dementia is something new. If they are laughing at inappropriate times and situations, if they laugh every time (or almost every time) you ask them a question, or if they laugh while making comments about not being able to remember something on a regular basis, you need to consider the possibility that your loved one is entering the world of dementia.

Dementia is no laughing matter, though, so don't ignore the signs and symptoms.

Take the initiative to gracefully and respectfully talk to your loved one about getting an examination that includes a memory evaluation and blood work to rule out infections, arterial disease, and other possible causes that can be treated promptly and sufficiently so that your loved one (and you) can enjoy many more years of making memories and having countless reasons to laugh with one another.

Are They Listening

Gerald was always a stickler for staying on top of home repairs and things like that. All I had to do was mention that something wasn't working exactly right, and he'd make sure to get it fixed. He wasn't the handiest of handymen, but he never hesitated to call someone who could.

I think that was my first clue that something wasn't right. I mentioned that the hot water wasn't as hot as it normally was. He didn't say anything. Four days later we had no hot water. He actually got upset with me for not telling him about it. I told him I thought we needed to have it looked at a few times each day. But each time he'd just brush it off.

Things went downhill from there. Within a couple of months, I had to write notes and pin them to the furniture and tape them to the door to remind him I'd gone to the store, or when I was in the basement doing laundry. Otherwise he'd panic and accuse me of trying to sneak off.

I'm not ashamed to tell you I spent a few hours crying and wondering why, after sixty-three years of a happy, loving marriage, it had to end like that. I'm also not ashamed to say I'm almost thankful he died of a heart attack before the dementia got worse.

At least when he died, he knew who I was and the last words he said to me were, "I love you, Bet. I always have and always will." ~Betty

If you are the caregiver or family member of someone who has a hearing impairment, I have a question for you: Do you ever wonder if your loved one is actually listening to you?

Have they asked the same question over and over and over again in a relatively short period of time? If so, have you wondered if they just aren't listening, or has their memory loss progressed to the point that they honestly don't remember asking that same question just seconds (literally) ago?

Or…what if they never actually heard you the first…or second…or third time?

What if the real issue is that they are hearing impaired?

Think about it--we know that part of the aging process includes hearing impairment. We also know it's one of those age-related things that people tend to take for granted. It's going to happen, so….

Instead of accepting it as a part of aging and ignoring it, I'm suggesting (Gasp!) that we accept it as a part of aging, and deal with it accordingly. Just like we do with arthritis and decreased vision.

Dealing with hearing loss doesn't always or automatically translate into hearing aids. It can often be alleviated with the simple act of cleaning out your loved ones' ears! No, seriously, it's true. "Ear hygiene", for lack of a better term, often goes by the wayside as we get older. Especially when getting older includes memory loss.

People with cognitive impairments tend to forget or ignore the need for yearly wellness exams. They 'save' their trips to the doctor for the big stuff, i.e. their pacemaker checks, the PET scans to make sure their cancer hasn't come back, glaucoma screenings, and so forth. Don't get me wrong;

going to the doctor for the 'big stuff' is essential. But when people focus on those things, the little things like making sure you can hear properly, or that wax buildup is not interfering with your hearing, tends to be ignored.

Whether they need a good cleaning or hearing aids— enhancing your loved one's ability to hear is generally not too difficult to do. It is usually a relatively easy fix with great big returns. That's why I want to encourage you to get your loved one's hearing evaluated. By doing all you can to ensure they are hearing at optimal level, they (and everyone around them) will be better able to enjoy talking and interacting with others.

That's not the only benefit to better hearing, though. Better hearing alleviates:

- Frustration and feeling left out
- Feeling ignored
- Feeling dumb for not knowing what's going on
- Feeling as if people are handling you
- Feeling disrespected and invisible

If these things are happening...

If you notice any of the following, take your loved one to the doctor for a hearing test/evaluation. Don't stop there, though. Follow up with whatever course of treatment the doctor recommends. Being able to hear is a quality of life you don't want your loved one to miss out on.

Here are a few signs your loved one may be experiencing which indicate hearing loss...

- The television volume is turned up excessively loud

- Repeatedly asking, "What?" "Huh?", or "I didn't catch that?
- Watching your lips intently why you talk
- Only responding to the questions or comments you make if they are facing you
- Being oblivious to the conversation going on around them
- Not participating in conversations that involve more than two people
- They stop listening to the television or radio
- They never talk about things they hear
- They withdraw from social gatherings

Dementia is a cruel disease. Don't add to the cruelty by adding to their burden of impaired hearing. We owe to our loved ones to do all we can to make their life as pleasant and stress-free as possible for as long as possible. Hearing is one of those things, so take my advice and help them hear. You'll all be better and happier for it.

When is it Time to Stop Driving

The day Wayne handed me the keys to the car and said he thought I'd better drive, was the day I knew life would never be the same.

A couple of weeks after he got out of a long stay in the hospital, he was going to drive down to our boat dock and check on the boats. He got in the car and...sat there. I saw him out the window and wondered what he was doing.

It took days for him to admit what had happened. He couldn't remember how to start the car.

My heart ached for him. I know how hard that was on his 'manly pride'. But I was also relieved that he had the wherewithal to admit when he was 'done'. I don't think he would have handled it well if I would have had to tell him he wasn't going to be able to drive.

These days he sits and sleeps most of the time. Or watches the lake while sitting on the deck. His short-term memory is completely gone, and his long-term memory is shaky at best. But we do okay. At least we can still smile, and he isn't too scared of my driving. ~Doris

"When it is time for a loved one to stop driving?", is a question I am frequently asked by family members of my patients. Notice I said family members, not the patients, themselves. There's a reason for that. In a word...INDEPENDENCE.

Driving is the superhero of independence. The coveted gold medal of growing up. The independence that comes with driving is unlike anything else. And for that reason, the question of when it's time to yank that independence away from someone is my least favorite question. Most of us started driving when we were teenagers, which translates into decades for most dementia patients. It is also not uncommon for these dear people to have unblemished records, i.e. not even a parking ticket to their name! Others have only a few minor mishaps on their record. Either way, almost without exception, each and every single one of these people will tell you they are a good driver. A safe driver. A conscientious driver. A driver in full possession of their faculties. In other words, drivers that do not need to relinquish this coveted form of independence.

Unfortunately, their impaired memories have diminished their driving ability without them realizing it. Everyone else, on the other hand, is keenly aware of these changes.

If asked about their driving ability, they'll tell you they're fine. And that may be true. They may not have had any traffic citations or accidents. They might possibly do fine as far as braking, accelerating, judging distance, following the speed limits, and even parallel parking. But are they safe? And are the people sharing the road with them safe? How fast are their reflexes and their response time? What happens in that split second when they have to make a decision because someone pulls out in front of them?

There's also the dilemma of whether or not they would admit getting lost or turned around in familiar locations. Failing to share this information is always for one of two reasons:

Reason one: They are afraid to tell you because they know if they do, you are going to take their keys away from them. Their driving days will be over and their independence, too.

Reason two: They don't remember to tell you because they don't remember it happening. And when or if they do remember, they are too scared to say anything because saying it makes it real.

From independent to isolated

Taking away driving privileges increases their level of isolation, which can then progress into a depression on top of the ever-worsening cognitive impairment. Remember— an elderly person doesn't have a houseful of kids, coworkers, or other opportunities to socialize the way we do when we're younger.

Eventually they will be a widow or widower, and their friends will be dying in rapid progression. Then when you factor in their inability to go anywhere without having to ask for a ride, their limitations and their despondency are greatly increased.

As a caregiver or family member, you need to be careful not to minimize or marginalize their feelings. Most people don't want to ask others to take them to the grocery store or to the shopping mall. They don't want to be a 'bother'. And a lot of people genuinely enjoy the actual activity of driving. So, to take this privilege away is...sad.

Making the call

Whenever I'm asked about driving privileges, my clinical response is to put safety first, and I advise you to do the same.

Safety—your loved one's and everyone else's—should be your number-one concern when thinking about whether or not your loved one should be driving.

- Do you feel safe when you are in the car with them?
- Would you let your young children ride with them?
- Do they have hearing difficulties?
- Do they still recognize the road signs?

Make no mistake about it—it's not an easy or comfortable conversation to have. It's not natural, for one thing, and the ramifications could be unpleasant. Upsetting your elderly parent by telling them they are a safety risk can cause problems in your relationship, but it's a risk you may well have to take. It may very well save the lives of your parent and of innocent people. Yes, safety must take top billing.

I know the time is coming (sooner rather than later) when I'm going to have to tell my mom driving is no longer an option for her. I am already a bit uneasy about riding with her, and I make sure she doesn't go very far or on busy, congested streets. So for now, we're good, but it's coming.

Making the call to put an end to your loved one's driving privileges needs to be done with a great sensitivity and respect. How you approach the matter can make the difference in how they receive and accept the news. I've been in on several of these conversations over the years, so I've seen it all. Some are disappointed but understand it's for the best. Even though they may not think it's necessary, they concede that they couldn't live with themselves if they hurt someone. Some people get defensive. Some get angry, and some sigh in resignation. And once in a while, you will find someone who actually comes to me (or their family members) first. They know it's time and want to be the one to make that decision instead of having it made for them.

I respect that. A lot. I can only imagine what it must feel like to realize you are no longer capable of doing something you've done for years. And done very well.

If you've decided the time has come, but know you are going to need help convincing your loved one the time to stop driving has come, you can always call on the doctor, other family members, or even your loved one's close friends to help you and your loved one put it in park for the last time and transition to this new phase of their life.

The Why of Vitamin B

Years ago, when you had a family doctor—a doctor who would sit and talk to you...and listen, our family doctored with Doc Myers. He didn't have all the fancy machines for testing this and that, and he didn't send you from one doctor to another who specializes in things. He listened to what you said was bothering or hurting you, asked questions, examined you, and then prescribed a treatment or medicine he thought would solve the problem. Most of the time it did.

One of the things he did for me was give me a vitamin B12 shot every month for my anemia. And if for some reason I missed it, you can believe I felt it. When he retired, his son took over the practice, and he continued the shots. But then he decided to move to a bigger city, and we were left to find a new doctor. Over the course of the next several years we went through 4 or 5 doctors. A couple of them dropped us because we were Medicare patients. Another one was just not nice, and the other one wanted to prescribe a pill for everything. But none of them—not even the doctor we finally felt comfortable with—would give me the B12 shot every month. Or ever, for that matter. They said it was a hoax and not even legal. My body begged to differ with them.

I settled for taking B12 supplements for several years, but every year when I had my physical, the blood work always came back showing I was anemic. The doctors would prescribe iron (which only caused worse constipation), folic acid, and once he even set up a series of blood transfusions that I cancelled. They also told me to stop drinking coffee and tea. Sorry, but one cup of coffee every morning and an occasional iced tea was not the problem. I tried to tell them, but they wouldn't listen.

Then along came Dr. Judy. She was an ear/nose/throat doctor and treated me for my thyroid cancer. After the surgery, she put me on some thyroid medication and then said we would have to really keep an eye on my anemia— something she noticed a history of on my records. I told her about the shots, and she said, "Those old-time docs knew what they were doing. We don't have all the answers and just because we don't know why something works doesn't mean it doesn't."

She went on to say that technically she couldn't administer the shot because it wasn't an approved treatment, but that she could prescribe the B12 if I wanted to do it myself or have my granddaughter do it. So, that's what we did. And wouldn't you know it—three months later I had my yearly physical, and the bloodwork didn't indicate I was anemic. ~Wanda

So, what's so special about vitamin B, or more specifically, the B complex vitamins?

The short answer is that they have an impact on the health of your brain and your cognitive abilities. But before we get into the details of that and the obvious reasons this is important to someone with dementia, I want to take a minute to explain why the B complex of vitamins is different and safer in terms of daily dosages.

Fact #1: all vitamins fall into one of two categories: fat-soluble or water-soluble.

Fat-soluble vitamins (A, D, E, and K) are stored in fat tissues where they hang out until you need them. The more you eat or ingest one of these supplements or foods rich in these vitamins, the more you have stored in your body. And because they have a 'shelf life' of up to six months, you can see how it might be possible to overload your system.

 For example, someone who ingests an excess of yellow veggies rich in vitamin A can actually start looking a bit orangish-yellow (skin tone).

Water-soluble vitamins, on the other hand (B), hang out in your body fluid. So, whenever you excrete body fluids (sweat, urine, stool), the vitamins leave with it. In other words, much of the talk about excess B12 in your system is unfounded...with exceptions, or course, because there are always exceptions to any 'rule'.

The exceptions to this rule apply to anyone who has impaired kidney function, those with certain eye and vision disorders and diseases, and people with excess iron in their system can experience negative side effects from having too much B12. Research has also been done, but is inconclusive, on the possible links between too much B12 and heart attacks and strokes. So...be sure you work with your healthcare professional to monitor your intake of B12 and the level of B12 in your system.

Okay, now that we've got that out of the way, let's talk B complex.

Facts:

- There are 8 vitamins in the B complex family
- Three of them play a significant role in cognitive function

- ○ B6 (pyridoxine)
- ○ B9 (folic acid)
- ○ B12 (cobalamin)
- Consistent and appropriate levels of the three cognitive related B complex vitamins in your system help slow cognitive decline and promote brain health

When I say they play a role in promoting brain health and cognitive abilities, what I mean is that they aid and promote the production of three important neurotransmitters. FYI: a neurotransmitter is a chemical in the brain which the brain uses to communicate with the rest of the body. The three chemicals (neurotransmitters) that I'm specifically talking about are serotonin, dopamine, and the one referred to as GABA.

- B6 is necessary in order to convert amino acids, which are also the building blocks of proteins, into neurotransmitters. The recommended daily dose of B6 is somewhere between 30 and 500 milligrams per day. But keep in mind that this recommended amount is for the average person. B6 can be found in several foods.
- B9, aka folic acid, is so important that many of the foods we buy are actually artificially fortified with folic acid. The number-one reason for the push in folic acid is due to the fact that it is proven to prevent neural tube defects in a fetus such as spina bifida. Folic acid is also a key component of all prenatal vitamins pregnant women are strongly encouraged to start taking as soon as they decide to try to get pregnant or become pregnant. The benefits of B9 are not solely reserved for pregnant

women and the unborn. It is also essential for a healthy immune system and energy production. There are many natural sources of B9; particularly green leafy vegetables, citrus fruits, and legumes. The recommended daily dose of B9 is 400 micrograms per day. Not milligrams. The abbreviation for micrograms is mcg.

- B12, also known as cobalamin, plays a vital role in nerve health. Oftentimes when people are deficient in B12, you start to notice brain fog or some memory issues. That's because B12 aids in nerve health, neuron (brain cells) health, and the production of red blood cells. FYI: Red blood cells carry oxygen throughout the body. The recommended daily dose of B12 is anywhere between, 400 micrograms and 2000 micrograms per day and can be found in meat, poultry, seafood, as well as fortified cereals.

B12 deficiencies

Because B12 is most closely related to the issue of dementia (neuron health and proper oxygen supply to the brain, and the rest of the body, as well), I want to spend some time explaining why adequate amounts of B12 are so important.

Let's start by looking at some of the basic causes of a B12 deficiency.

1: Pernicious anemia, which is what Wanda had. Someone with pernicious anemia cannot absorb B12 in their gut (stomach). This means the B12 they take orally, either by way of foods or supplements, does little to no good. And that is why Wanda needed the monthly injections. Her 'old time' doc took the time to discern the type of anemia Wanda had, whereas the other doctors went by a few numbers on a bloodwork panel and called it good.

If your B12 intake and absorption rate is low, you will most likely experience fatigue weakness, and even shortness of breath. Some people even notice numbness in their extremities. Shortness of breath and numbness in someone's extremities can be caused by other factors but if you or your loved one is experiencing this, an evaluation including checking a B12 level is certainly warranted.

The balance disturbance that comes from numbness in their feet and even their hands, puts them at a greater risk for falling.

Falls, as we know, are fatal, more often than not, in one way or another among the elderly, so whatever we can do to help them avoid falling, should be done. Including checking for B12 deficiency and remedying it.

B12 deficiency is determined by a simple blood test. B12 is not always on the bloodwork panel that's ordered. Unless you report something to indicate to your healthcare provider that it needs to checked, it likely won't be. So as an advocate for your loved one, insist on having it checked.

There's another test called a homocysteine level that can be done. Homocysteine is a byproduct of digestion, and B12 helps to clear it. When their B12 is low, the homocysteine levels will increase, because it has an inverse relationship. This is also something you'd want to talk to your healthcare provider about.

Another group of people that tend to be at risk of B12 deficiency are individuals who are on special diets. For example, vegetarians and vegans are at a particularly increased risk of a B12 deficiency because of the fact that B12 is consumed by eating foods (primarily meat) that vegetarians and vegans don't eat.

Two other groups of people whose ability to absorb B12 is compromised or even impossible are:

- Those who have had gastric bypass. People who've had gastric bypass do not have the ability to absorb B12 through their gut; meaning they will require B12 injections for the rest of their life.
- The elderly. The problem with the elderly is the aging process—the natural deterioration of the body slows and eventually resists the absorption of B12 by the body.

Drug interactions

Certain medications (prescription and OTC) interrupt or prohibit the absorption of B12. This is something few people outside the medical profession think about. But that doesn't make it any less a problem, and since you are your loved one's best advocate, I believe it is important to provide you with a list of medications that fall under this category. NOTE: Some of these are not relevant to the elderly, but since knowledge is power…

- Excessive amounts of ibuprofen
- Oral contraceptives
- Colchicine (gout treatment)
- Tagamet
- Prilosec
- Phenobarbital
- Pregabalin (Lyrica)

- Primidone (Mysolin)
- Metformin

PLEASE NOTE: None of these greatly reduce or interfere with the body's B12 absorption abilities, but if someone is already not getting enough (for one reason or another), any interference can exasperate the problem. Therefore, I strongly suggest you stay on top of things by requesting your loved one's yearly blood work include a B12 test. Furthermore, if you notice the warning signs of B12 deficiency, you would not be out of line to request the test at any time.

Neurotransmitters and B complex vitamins

Let's talk about serotonin. When people hear the word 'serotonin, they think about depression, and anxiety, because serotonin keeps our moods balanced. Low serotonin contributes to anxiety and depression, which in turn, can lead to poor memory function and can possibly lead to Alzheimer's.

Serotonin levels can be raised significantly by exercise. Good, old-fashioned physical exercise. You also need to know/remember that serotonin produces endorphin chemicals.

Endorphins are often referred to as the body's feel-good or happy chemicals. So, let's put this all together to see what we've got:

EXERCISE makes SEROTONIN. SEROTONIN produces ENDORPHINS. ENDORPHINS boost our mood.

The moral of this story is EXERCISE.

The next neurotransmitter on our list is dopamine. Dopamine regulates mood as well as muscle movement.

Dopamine deficiencies at their worst result in Parkinson's disease. Parkinson's robs its victim of muscle movement, speech, memory, and all other cognitive abilities to the point of death.

Schizophrenia is another horrible disease caused by dopamine. But it isn't a dopamine deficiency, that causes schizophrenia. It's just the opposite—extreme excess amounts of dopamine.

But dopamine is not normally problematic. Quite the contrary! In the vast majority of people, dopamine plays a vital role in the brain's ability to understand and experience pleasure.

We all want to experience pleasurable experiences of all kinds, so it behooves us to make sure we maintain a healthy level of dopamine in our system. And in our loved one's system.

How do we do that? Exercise! That's right—once again, exercise is the answer. Exercise promotes the production of dopamine, while at the same time working to slow down the rate at which brain cells die off.

Dopamine also plays an important part in keeping our working memory (short term) healthy, our ability to reason, and to make sound decisions.

Finally, let's talk about GABA. GABA is an inhibitory neurotransmitter, which means it calms you. GABA is important with respect to memory because it helps to promote cognitive focus. GABA helps you relax and stay focused on what you are learning what you're listening to, what memories you're trying to create. It can actually even cause you to feel somewhat sedated if you have an excess of this neurotransmitter in your system.

GABA levels are increased by our consumption of whole grains, nuts, including walnuts, and almonds and sunflower seeds, shrimp, and halibut. Most berries and cocoa are also good choices for raising your GABA level.

There's a reason it's called B complex

It would be impossible to miss the message that the B complex vitamins are extremely valuable to our health. Literally from our head (brain) to our toes (keeping the nerves in our feet stimulated and appropriately sensitive). They're all interconnected. For this reason, I strongly suggest talking to your healthcare professional about adding a B complex supplement to your daily regimen. I also suggest taking a proactive and keen interest in watching for signs and symptoms of deficiencies of B vitamins.

I say this because my father, who I only see once or twice a year, seemed 'off' during some of our weekly phone conversations. Long story short, I was able to direct him to ask his doctor to test his B12 level. Turns out it was extremely low—low enough that the doctor bluntly informed my 80-year-old father that there was still time to turn this around. BUT…if he didn't, he was headed straight for a life of dementia.

Turns out my dad, who had always been a meat-lover, was trying to lose some weight, so had cut back drastically on foods rich in B12. He started getting injections, which has helped tremendously, and I have no doubt he will be able to transition to an oral supplement soon. Along with going back to eating more animal-based foods.

Had I not been in touch with what was normal for Dad, I wouldn't have noticed the downward spiral. And the moral of this story is BE LOVED ONE AWARE.

Understanding Long Term Memory

I watched my wife tirelessly and patiently care for Granny for several years. And whenever possible or feasible, I did what I could to help, too. Granny's Alzheimer's took a lot away from her—including her short-term memory. But it never robbed this amazing woman of her heart—a heart that loved more completely and unconditionally than anyone else I've ever come in contact with. I think that's why it was so easy to be unphased by the twenty-two million times a day she would repeat the same thing over and over and over again. Never ever did my wife act the least bit frustrated or irritated with Granny. She acted as if each question or comment was the first and only of its kind.

When I think about it just now, it's obvious that Granny's ability to love was transferred to my wife—that she was loving Granny back the way Granny always loved her.

Nobody wants dementia. Nobody wants to even think about the possibility that they might someday be where Granny was. But if I am, I know without a doubt that I'll be in good and loving hands, and that my lack of short-term memory won't be an irritation or frustration to my wife. Thanks, Granny, for that, and so much more. ~JW

Do you ever wonder why someone would forget what they had for breakfast, yet be able to tell you without skipping a beat, who their best friend was way back in third grade? And what they wore to their junior/senior prom?

 It's because what they had for breakfast is stored in their short-term memory bank, and the details from their childhood and teen years is in their long-term memory bank.

The brain's memory storage mechanisms are two vastly different 'machines' which are located in two different parts of the brain. And for reasons unknown, the short-term memory bank is the first victim of this dreadful disease. Likewise, the long-term memory is the last thing to go.

Short-term memory is defined as memories stored for 30 seconds up to several days. Dementia's effects on the short-term memory bank is why one of the first signs of dementia, especially Alzheimer's, is the constant repetition during a conversation. Long-term memory, however, is stored for a lifetime.

Short-term memories are things like what you eat for breakfast, who called to chat, what the doctor told them to do for their slipped disc, and or whether or not they wrote out a check for the utility bill this month.

Long-term memories are what give us the ability to know how to brush our teeth, drive a car, or who your best friend was when you were in third grade.

Since we know that short-term memory is going to be the first thing to go, I personally feel that focusing on nurturing and protecting long-term memory is most beneficial to the dementia patient. The psychology behind this is simple—when they don't have to deal with the frustration of what they can't remember, they are more confident and strive harder to hold on to what they can remember.

Two facets of long-term memory

The two facets of long-term memory are explicit long-term memory and implicit long-term memory. Explicit memory covers memories of facts and experiences. An example of semantic memory would be that the United States is part of North America (fact), and which parts of the United States they have traveled to (experience).

Implicit memory is the automatic type of memory. It's the memory that involves motor movement, i.e. how to walk, how to use a spoon, which hand you write with, and so on.

The crossover between long and short-term memory

Long-term memory:

- Knowing how to drive a car
- Knowing how to brush your teeth

Short-term memory:

- Forgetting what a stop sign is or how you got from your house to the market
- Not remembering if you brushed your teeth after breakfast

This crossover can be very confusing and frustration to people—both the one with dementia and their caregivers. They don't understand why they can remember some things but not others. But rather than focus on what you or your loved one can't remember, use what they can remember to add to the quality of their life.

When your loved one has advanced stage of any type of dementia, you need to make the conscious effort to tap into their long-term memory. Talk about the past. Play music that would be significant to their past. Surround them with tangible reminders of their past. These things will bring back fond memories and make them feel secure and validated, which after all, is exactly what we want for them, right? Absolutely!

Covid-19 and Dementia

Bob has Alzheimer's. Linda, his wife, has been caring for him in their home for the past three years. They have two grown children who are both involved and attentive to their parents' needs. But when Linda and Bob both contracted COVID-19 from the home healthcare worker who visits twice a week to give Bob some extra attention, their lives were turned upside down. Literally, overnight.

Linda spent weeks in the hospital—three days of which she was in critical condition. She was released a few days ago but will need several weeks of rest and a stress-free environment to get her strength back. The doctors and the kids have made it clear, however, that Bob will need to go to a fulltime care facility. COVID-19 caused his condition to take a nosedive, to the point that he is non-verbal and has little voluntary or controlled movement. Naturally, this doesn't make for a very stress-free environment for Linda. She is afraid Bob is looking for her and doesn't understand why she 'deserted' him.

It's such a sad situation. We all knew the day was coming when Linda wouldn't be able to care for Bob at home, but as her sister, I know how important it was to her to be a loving, devoted wife for better or worse…in sickness and in health. ~Judy

Who could have imagined just a few months ago, that our current pandemic COVID-19 could have such a rippling effect into absolutely every aspect of our life and our world? I know I certainly couldn't. But not being able to imagine it doesn't change the fact that COVID-19 has changed the world as we know it. And, unfortunately, from everything I can tell and from what I hear from the experts, the world we used to know, may be nothing more than a memory.

The present and the future are on the trajectory to consist of a new normal; something the youngest generation and future generations will only know as normal (nothing new about it).

I can't say that COVID-19 has had a significant impact on the number of memory evaluations I've done, but one thing I can say is this: COVID-19 has dramatically increased the number of patients I see and treat for depression. People who otherwise didn't have any kind of memory impairment, now find themselves struggling to remember simple things, and who are having difficulty finding the words they need to express their thoughts and feelings, and who are just having a tough time getting through the day.

As for those people who had been diagnosed with some type of cognitive impairment prior to the pandemic, they are now on an even more precipitous decline. And upon investigation and examination, this downward spiral can be attributed to the ramifications of COVID-19, i.e. social distancing, quarantining, avoidance of personal contact, and out and out fear.

People who prior to the pandemic, didn't have any significant cognitive impairment beyond normal age-related forgetfulness, are now struggling. I attribute this to the isolation guidelines and mandates that have been pushed upon us. It's not normal! It goes against our instincts and our comfort zones. It's so abnormal to us that it is having a huge negative impact on our bodies and our brains. Our physical health and our personality. Our mental state and our ability to be relational and communicative.

We aren't getting the type or amount of brain stimulation we're used to getting…the stimulation we've thrived on and prospered in for centuries. In the few months we've been isolated and not been in a position to visit, i.e. recall thoughts, beliefs, and facts in order to discuss them with other people, and we are forgetting them. I'll also take the opportunity here to reiterate the increased numbers of people experiencing depression and anxiety, which only make memory problems worse.

Fortunately, we can treat these problems by eliminating them to the greatest possible extent. We need to stop isolating people from each other. We need to make concerted efforts to communicate using a number of different mediums in order to stimulate the different parts of the brain. We can increase the amount of exercise they get, offer activities that 'force' them to think, reason, make logical deductions, and choices, and to use both short and long-term memory. And you know what? With little to no exceptions, their situation (memory) improves.

For those who came into the world of COVID-19 already burdened with cognitive impairment issues, things aren't as easy, and the outcome isn't as positive or 'rosy'. Instead of trying to backpaddle (reverse the damage), the best we can do is work hard to manage the new symptoms as effectively as possible so that we can hopefully put the brakes on their rapid decline.

Even those dementia patients who can't comprehend the seriousness of the situation, still have the ability (much of the time, anyway) to perceive anxiety and stress. They are surrounded by it. Family members, their caregivers, their healthcare workers, and everyone else they have any form of contact with, send out "COVID-19" vibes, because no one can go through a single day without being affected by it in some way or another.

Quite honestly, it's taking a toll on everybody. Young or old, rich or poor, rural or city dweller, white collar or blue collar…no matter who you are, you are up to your eyeballs in COVID19 information, misinformation, and everything in between.

No matter what you think about it, or how seriously you view the situation, this fact remains: it's here to stay, at least for now, so somehow we have to find a way to break the cycle of what it's doing to our elderly loved ones. We have to stop letting it deteriorate and destroy what quality of life they have left.

How? How are we going to do that?

Sorry, I don't have any firm answers to that. I'm asking a rhetorical question because we have to come up with an answer. If we don't the problems with how COVID-19 is affecting our mental and emotional health are only going to get worse. There will be an upswing in cases of people suffering from various forms of dementia. We will become a society of mentally and emotionally dysfunctional people.

If you are like me, which I think most of you are, you aren't expecting a crystal-ball kind of clarity and revealing as to what is going to happen in the future. You know that's not possible. But what you DO want for yourself and your loved one is the go-ahead to make the most of the new normal guidelines and make them work for you. Adapt them to the capabilities and limitations of your loved one for maximum benefit. For example, make the most of outdoor activities by creating socialization and relational interaction that fall within the perimeters of what is allowed and deemed safe. Get creative with how you increase the levels of physical, emotional, and mental exercise in their day to day activities. Stop being non-social and stop denying your loved one from being social. Just do it differently. But make sure 'different' includes conversation, sharing of opinions, ideas, and memories.

I also want to strongly suggest you stop the flow of information/misinformation overload. My friends, you don't have to look far to find someone who will tell you what you want to hear. The trouble with this is that what you want to hear isn't always what you need to hear. Nor is it always the truth. This information overload is also stressful on our memories and our state of mind.

I'm not recommending you bury your head in the sand. But I am suggesting you stop focusing on COVID-19 24/7 and start focusing on what is good in this world AND how to make a bad situation better—lemonade out of lemons, if you will. We don't have the ability to stop COVID-19. Nor do we have the ability to change the way the world is handling it. But what we do have the ability to do, is control how WE handle or deal with it, and how our attitude bleeds over into the care of our loved ones— especially those with dementia.

Remember: What wears you down makes you sad, so do something positive. Something that makes you happy. Likewise, do the same for your loved one. Their quality of life (and yours) is counting on you.

Surgery, Anesthesia, and Dementia…

What You Need to Know

I was fourteen when my youngest sister had her tonsils out. That was almost twenty years ago, but I can still remember two things about that day as clearly as if it were yesterday. I remember how scared I was when she first started waking up from the anesthesia. She was so disoriented. She didn't know where she was and when I said, "Hey, Em, it's me," she said she didn't know me. The second thing I remember is everything she said after that for the next hour—and how hard we laughed because it was so funny.

A couple of years later, though, our elderly neighbor who had dementia, and who I was close to, had to have hernia surgery. Knowing what I knew even as a teenager, about dementia, I was worried about Earl and what the anesthesia would do to him. It wasn't pretty. Instead of a couple of hours of confusion, it was a couple of days of being more disoriented and confused than normal. It was so sad. And in my opinion, the dementia got worse at a faster rate after that. I know that might sound like I'm trying to find excuses or whatever, but from what I've learned since then, I think it's true. I know Linda (his daughter) didn't have a choice in the matter, but I think the medical profession should work hard to find a way to treat dementia patients for things like that in a way that won't take what little they have left of themselves any sooner than it has to be. ~Olivia

This young lady is right. Post-surgical memory impairment does decline more rapidly. Research proves it. But it's a 'catch 22', because let's face it—the senior population is the group with the greatest needs for surgery of any kind—planned or emergency. So, when you put the two together, it's like mixing baking soda and vinegar. Trouble bubbles up and spills over into everything in its path. That's why, as the caregiver and/or loved one of a dementia patient, you need to be equipped with as much knowledge and information as possible, so that you can have a plan in place for how to deal with the situation when it arises.

Planned surgery

First let's talk about planned surgery. You know, things like hip or knee replacements, oral surgery, and things of that nature. When you have your surgical consultation with the doctor, you need to find out whether or not it is a general anesthesia type of surgery or if the procedure could be done with a spinal block or local anesthesia. And here's why…

General anesthesia takes a while to clear the system—much longer than after waking up in the recovery room. Oftentimes, it takes several weeks for it to leave the body completely. And during that time, the lingering anesthesia has a cognitive impact. The person's memory remains a bit foggy, and unfortunately doesn't bounce back to what it was before they had general anesthesia. Therefore, what I recommend, especially for planned surgeries, is to ask what your options for anesthesia are. You might be surprised to find out that in many cases, you can request to have a spinal block or a local anesthesia.

FYI: A spinal block is a procedure that injects medication capable of numbing the body into the spine. It lasts only a few hours, and the patient remains awake and alert. A local anesthesia works similarly, except the anesthesia is injected into the area surrounding the location of the procedure and numbs just that portion of the body.

Unfortunately, there are some surgeries where general anesthesia is the only type that you can have. Bypass surgery or lung surgeries being two examples of that. Emergency procedures usually require general anesthesia, too. The primary reason for that, is the inability to plan ahead. Emergencies don't give us that 'luxury'.

Another discussion you need to have prior to a planned surgery is the discussion with the anesthesiologist. It is important that they are aware of the fact that the person they will be administering the medication to, has cognitive/memory impairment. Conditions such as these actually determine how much medication a patient receives and at what rate they receive it. Because medications such as these (as well as others) are metabolized differently in people with cognitive/memory impairment, this affects not only how they respond to the medication going into the surgery, but how they respond coming out from under the effects. In other words, it affects how they wake up in the recovery room (the length of time it takes, their personality, and so forth).

Beyond telling the doctor, surgeon, and anesthesiologist, the nurses and aides who will be caring for your loved one also need to be made aware of their condition. I said in the last chapter that information is power when it comes to dealing with COVID-19, but that statement is equally true in this case, too. The more information caregivers have about their patients, the better care they can give them.

Unplanned surgery

I've already alluded to the fact that the majority of unplanned surgeries will require general anesthesia. The necessity of general anesthesia, however, does NOT negate or reduce the level of importance you should place on having the conversations we just talked about with the care team—from the surgeon and anesthesiologist, to the nurses and the aides responsible for supplying post-op ice chips and warm blankets.

It's quite possible that the conversations will be a bit more rushed and that you won't be able to fully explain what stage their dementia is at, but you need to make sure they know who they are treating and what they are dealing with. Failing to make these facts known is unfair to your loved one AND the caregivers. A medical professional has taken an oath to give the highest quality of care and respect to every patient that comes their way. They can't offer those things to your loved one if they don't know what added risk factors are involved.

When to be concerned

Let's say your loved one had to have general anesthesia and you have noticed their increased level of impairment doesn't seem to be getting any better. Should you contact the doctor? Should you work with your loved one to try to regain their former level of clarity? Or should you just accept the new normal and go forward as is?

I like to tell my patients and their families to give it several weeks before getting concerned that you've arrived at a new normal. It really can take that long. Just be aware, take notes, and try not to let your loved one know how concerned you are. Their added disorientation is enough stress for them to have to deal with. And as always, don't hesitate to call your healthcare team to discuss your concerns and to get answers to your questions. It's what we're here for.

Please know, as we get ready to move on to the next topic, that I am in no way suggesting you should refuse general anesthesia for your loved one or put off surgical procedures requiring general anesthesia. Not at all! I just want you to be aware of the possible options available in many cases that can make surgical procedures less traumatic, less invasive, and less apt to push the 'decline button' of their cognitive impairment.

As always, it's about quality of life. If quality means general anesthesia to correct a problem, then that's what you need to do. But if quality means taking an easier route, then by all means, do so.

Self-Esteem and Dementia

The first time I had to clean my grandma's bowel movement off the chair and the floor leading to the bathroom, I honestly can't tell you who cried more—me or her. She cried because in her words, "You shouldn't have to be doing that for me. I'm not living, I'm just existing, so I wish God would just take me." I cried because I felt so bad for her. She knew what had happened and it was a major blow to her self-esteem and her modesty. But instead of letting her feel that way, I held her tight and said, "I don't have to do this for you. I get to. I get to take care of you just like you've always taken care of me. It's my turn now, Granny, and I'm honored to be the one who does." ~Darla

How do you measure your own success? Most men measure their success by their career achievements and the dollar amount in their bank account. Women, on the other hand, tend to measure success by the way their family reflects back on them.

The question of measuring success might seem like a strange question to ask, but consider this: Have you ever wondered how your loved one with dementia feels about his/herself? We know that depression is common in senior citizens in general, but it is even more prevalent in the population of seniors with dementia. Think about it—they are socially isolated (even beyond what has been brought on by the pandemic), they are unable (or at least less able) to communicate logically or participate in conversations without feeling confused. What's more, because they are no longer gainfully employed, and because their family is grown and long-gone from needing the type of care and attention they once did, an elderly person's 'success measuring rod' is gone. Oh, and then on top of all that, when you add in the fact that they are often dependent on other people for some of life's most basic needs....

Well, you can see where I'm going with this, right? It doesn't take a genius to figure out that putting all that together makes it incredibly easy for low self-esteem and depression to take root and grow in the hearts and minds of our senior citizens.

Just because it's easy doesn't make it right, though, which is where we come in. As loved ones and caregivers, we need to make sure we are doing all we can to promote a strong sense of self-esteem, self-worth, and sense of success in those who are struggling with memory impairment so that they can feel good about themselves. Here is what I suggest:

#1: Don't talk for them or do for them anymore than is ABSOLUTELY necessary. You obviously need to provide assistance when it is needed, and as always, safety should be kept at the forefront of everything they do, but anytime you can promote their self-esteem through being self-reliant and independent (even in the little things) you need to do so.

#2: Allow these individuals to live independently for as long as possible. Even if living independently requires you to monitor their financial activities, have groceries delivered, and so forth, the independence of aging in place (staying in their own home) for as long as possible is enormously important to their self-esteem.

#3: Don't set them up for failure by expecting too much. To help you in this regard, I want to encourage you to use what

I call the "One Step Command Technique". It's super-easy. As easy as One. That's it—just one.

Here's how it works: Give your loved one just one instruction at a time. Instead of saying, "Would you mind scraping the plates, put them in the dishwasher, and put the leftovers in the refrigerator?" Just as say, "Would you please scrape the plates into the garbage can for me?"

Someone with short-term memory impairment can't remember three things. They just can't. But when you give them three things to do, and they only do one, often times we respond with something like, "Why aren't the plates in the dishwasher?" "Have you put the plates in the dishwasher yet?" "Don't forget to take care of the leftovers. We don't want to waste them."

See the differences? Do you see why giving more than one command can make them feel like a failure? Even though they don't necessarily remember you giving them the other two, your comments insinuate they should remember, or plant seeds of doubt in their minds that they didn't do what you wanted them to. These thoughts lead to poor self-esteem, a lack of confidence, sadness, and depression.

By providing a one-step command, you are promoting their self-esteem and making them feel useful. They justifiably believe that they can still contribute to the family and to society. And isn't that what everyone wants? We all want to feel as though we contribute. That we participate in our life, and we make the lives of those around us better by helping. By giving vs. only receiving. And once again, I ask: Isn't that what everyone wants?

Yes. Yes, it is.

You need to understand that dementia knows no boundaries. It doesn't matter what your socioeconomic background is, what level of education you have achieved, what your last name is, what the color of your skin is, what your religious beliefs are, how many children you have, the square footage of your house, the number of stamps in your passport...none of this matters. None of these things matter when it comes to needing and wanting to feel useful, either. It's human nature to need to be needed. So, take the simple advice you've just been given to heart. Use it to enhance the lives of you and your loved one suffering with dementia so that you can all enjoy the benefits of knowing you are both valued and valuable. Because you are. We all are.

What Motivates You to Derail Dementia

I know Parkinson's disease is rarely hereditary. Trust me—after watching my dad's life slowly slip away because of it—I did a lot of reading and research to determine how at risk me and my adult sons were for going down this same path. If the possibilities were significant, I wanted to be prepared—as best I could, anyway. But even knowing it's not hereditary, I am so much more aware of the pain and heartache any form of dementia brings to a person and their family. As a preacher, I've spent countless hours praying with families beside hospital beds, in nursing homes, and in their homes. Praying for God to mercifully release a loved one from their pain. Praying for strength and courage for those caring the person they love, but who no longer even knows their name. It's not easy. It stinks. And even though I know God's ways are perfect and that he knows what is best, I am still doing my part to treat my body as his temple, so that hopefully I and my family are spared the disease called dementia. ~Dave

What motivates you to do the things you do? More specifically, and because of the subject matter of this book, what motivates you to try to deter or ward off dementia? For me, the answer to that question is fear.

Part of my fear comes from my family's history of dementia. Part of my fear comes from my chosen career path. I am surrounded by the realities and uncertainties that are dementia. Because of these things, I'm going to do everything I possibly can do to delay or hopefully even avoid it altogether. Or at the very least, I am going to

105

educate my loved ones and everyone else I can on the realities of dementia, so that if or when I am 'there', I will benefit from their knowledge and understanding of my needs and the journey I am taking.

At this point I am going to say that if you are reading this, chances are you have these very same feelings and concerns. Why? Because either you are dealing with the realities of dementia in your family right now, or you have done so in the past. You know (as well as anyone can who isn't actually living the nightmare) what dementia does to its victim and their loved ones.

So, when I ask you what motivates you, it's really my way of saying, stop putting off for tomorrow (or next week…month…year) what you can do today and every day. Stop wasting time. Starting right now, stop letting fear stand between you and making each day better. Starting today, do at least one thing to make your brain healthier and keep it that way.

Don't make excuses such as not having time or needing to wait until this or that project or stage of life is done. Don't wait, because dementia is one of the many things that genuinely benefits from the mindset (no pun intended) that an ounce of prevention really is worth a pound of cure.

Dementia begins looooooooong before there are any symptoms or clinical signs it is there. You don't just wake up one morning to discover that your short-term memory is impaired. It's happening behind the scenes long before you 'suddenly' can't remember the names of your great grandkids or miss a doctor's appointment because it slipped your mind. And while paranoia is definitely not something you want to add to your list of things you are good at, you also don't want to live in a state of denial by using the excuse that your impaired memory is just part of getting old.

We have to be proactive without being paranoid. We have to assume we are at risk because the reality is that we are. Every single one of us is at risk for some type of dementia. Even if you don't have any family members that have dementia. You, too, are at risk because the number one greatest risk factor for developing some type of dementia is age. That is why I am taking a break in this chapter from talking about your loved ones, and instead, want to talk about you. I want to challenge you to take control of your life. Recognize that you're in the driver's seat when it comes to caring for your body and your mind.

No, you can't control whether or not you get dementia at some point in your life. But what you can do is work toward lowering your risk factors by:

- Getting plenty of exercise
- Eating a healthy diet
- Avoiding tobacco
- Limiting your intake of alcohol
- Getting the proper amount of rest you need each night
- Stimulating your brain through reading, hobbies, games, puzzles, conversation, socialization, educational experiences (seminars, museums, etc.)
- Healthy relationships with family and friends
- Getting regular checkups to prevent unexpected health emergencies like heart attacks and strokes, which often lead to vascular dementia

- Be a positive person—limit or better yet, eliminate the stress factors in your life
- Educate yourself on the various forms of dementia and be mindful of any symptoms and signs
- Take action if you notice these signs and symptoms by getting tested (better safe than sorry)

I've had health scares over the years involving myself, my husband, my kids, and my parents. They're no fun, to say the least. But then you probably already know that, too, don't you?

So, whether it be fear, the memories of those health scares, or whatever else you consider motivating, take it to heart. BE MOTIVATED to take action starting today. Be motivated to make today the day you take action to keep dementia from taking action against you.

When Home No Longer Seems Like Home

When my mom was in the final stages of Alzheimer's she spent each day believing she was a nine-year-old girl going to school, winning a spelling bee, and playing with her friends. She recognized one person and one person only— her great grandson, Zach. Zach was eight at the time. My nephew and niece in-law (Zach's parents) did a wonderful job helping Zach understand why Grandma Ruth said the things she said and did the things she did, so it didn't upset him when she would ask him to play, or ask him to help her find something because it wasn't where she'd left it.

It wasn't there because in her mind, she still lived with my grandparents and aunt. This home...her home for the last forty years, wasn't a place she recognized. With people she didn't recognize. Except Zach. I can't lie—it wasn't easy being in the room with my mom knowing she didn't have a clue as to who I was. As far as she was concerned, I didn't exist—not as her daughter, anyway. How could I? In her mind she was a child.

It was also not uncommon for her to ask for her parents or why this or that in the house looked different. I usually gave her a quick, nonchalant answer like, "I don't know," or "It looks nice, doesn't it?" Or I would answer with another question like, "Do you like it?" or "What do you mean?". At that point, the best we could do was take one day or even hour at a time and just roll with it. ~Barbara Jo

If your loved one is in an advanced stage of dementia, you have undoubtedly heard them say something along the lines of, "I want to go home," a few (hundred) times. Or if not that, they question where they are...and possibly who you are.

It can be quite frustrating and sad for you, while at the same time, it is frustrating and even quite unsettling for them. But then, that's dementia. Frustrating, sad, unsettling, and just plain awful.

Every once in a while, I come across a family member who is uncertain of what their loved one means when they talk about going home. They ask me to explain what their loved one means or is asking for. This is especially true when it's a new phase or if there is nothing to accompany their request such as talking about their siblings, their parents, or a landmark or event from their childhood you know about.

To make matters even worse, sometimes, because it throws you off guard, your response may be something like, "You are home," or "This is your house—you've lived here fifty years, don't you remember?" To which they respond by becoming even more confused, agitated, or even scared. It's never as simple as just, "Oh, okay".

That is why you need to understand that more often than not, the home they are referring to is their home from the past. They no longer recognize their current surroundings nor accept them as the place they belong—no matter how long they've been there. You also need to understand how you need to respond and deal with this situation—for your own good as well as theirs.

The first thing I would tell you is not to challenge them. Your job, remember, as their caregiver and/or loved one is to reassure them that they are safe and loved. Not add to their confusion by telling them they are wrong. Think about it, what if someone told you that you were home, but you didn't recognize anything in the room. But anytime you questioned it, they insisted they were right, and you were wrong. Wouldn't you become anxious and scared?

The second piece of advice I have for you, is to distract them. For example, you could say, "I know you do, and we will...tomorrow. I still have some things I need to do here." Or "We will, as soon as we can."

Thirdly, encourage them to talk about the home they want to go back to. Guide the conversation so that you can learn more about 'home' and what makes it so special to them.

- Is it a special blanket or something about the room they slept in?
- Does he/she miss always smelling Mom's chicken pie or bread baking? Or the smell of their dad's pipe tobacco?
- The sounds of the chickens clucking and the rooster crowing?
- His/her mom's flower garden?
- A big tree they used to climb and hang out it?
- A special toy, such as a doll or a bb gun?
- The bright green aluminum cup they used to drink from?

Once you find out a few of these things, recreate them. To the extent that you can, anyways. For example:

- Get a similar blanket, redecorate their room to be more childlike, or to resemble what they remember.
- Candles come in all sorts of scents if you aren't into baking bread or smoking a pipe. Keep one lit to help them relish their memories and be at peace. BE SURE TO KEEP IT OUT OF THEIR REACH.

- Sound machines are not just for babies. There are free apps for your phone, your tablet, e-reader, or home 'guru' (google, alexa, etc.).
- Plant a flower garden or get some indoor plants. Or splurge on a few fresh-cut flowers in a vase each week for them to enjoy.
- No, don't let them climb a tree, but putting a lawn chair under a big shade tree and settling them into it for a couple of hours a day (weather permitting) would do wonders for their physical, emotional, mental, and spiritual wellbeing.
- Give them a toy or two from their past. Let them hold it, keep it near them, or even play with it.
- Vintage is in! You can find replicas of old dishes and household items for very little money. Buy a few to make them feel like they truly are home.

You will be amazed at how well these things work—both distracting them and incorporating things from home back into their lives. The reason these things work so well is because they tap into long-term memory, which is what they hold on to the longest.

Last but not least, be ready. You know by now that there is nothing you can do to stop the progression of this disease, so you know the day is coming when you are going to have to deal with this sort of thing. It's inevitable. That is why I strongly recommend that you be aware and prepared. When you notice that your loved one is starting to talk about loved ones, in particular, their parents, who probably are deceased, in present tense, you need to start moving toward making home a place they recognize and feel comfortable and safe in. You will know that at this point in time, the past is their present, which means it's time for you to give them back some of their past, so that their present and what future they have left, will be as meaningful and peaceful as it can possibly be.

Menopause, Memory, and Dementia

When I started experiencing some short-term memory issues, I panicked. Part of the reason I panicked because some of the things I forgot were significant. Like my granddaughter's school program. I had never done anything like that in my life! But the big reason for hitting the panic button was the visions I had of ending up like both of my grandmothers. Both had Alzheimer's and died in their early eighties because of it. My mom died in a car accident when I was twenty, so I don't know if she would have ended up that way. Thankfully, my dad, who is in his seventies, is fine. So, I know there's hope.

Anyway, I went to the doctor because I thought if I got a handle on it early, maybe, just maybe, I could put off the inevitable. As it turns out, I am entering menopause. Or I was. I'm smack dab in the middle of it. I still have some short-term memory issues, but I'm dealing with it without the added burden of panic and paranoia.

I know this isn't any guarantee I won't have dementia in the future. But here's something else I know—I know I'm going to do whatever I can to take care of myself now to try to keep myself as healthy as I can, because a healthy me now, can help to be a healthier me later on. I am especially focused on doing things to keep my mind sharp and alert. I guess you could say I exercise my brain every day to keep it in good shape. ~Joan

I'm just going to take a wild guess and say any woman who's either perimenopausal or menopausal understands that it is very common for women in these phases of life to experience memory difficulties similar to the type of memory issues that women who are in the early stages of Alzheimer's. You know—short-term memory issues, difficulty finding the right word, and even a bit of a recall problem.

These things aren't surprising to those with a medical background because what we know is that estrogen, the primary hormone involved in perimenopause and menopause, decreases during this time in a woman's life. And with it, comes a decrease in short-term memory. That's a broad statement, though, so let's break it down a little further.

First of all, let's make sure we understand the difference between perimenopause and menopause. During perimenopause, as estrogen levels start to decline, the menstrual cycle becomes irregular, and a woman may have a slight problem with memory issues. But as you are approaching the latter stage of perimenopause and entering menopause, you have a significant decline in your estrogen level, the menstrual cycle ceases, and short-term memory issues become even more of an issue. But why?

What we know about memory as it relates to estrogen is that it is linked to the estradiol form of estrogen. The job of estradiol is to create memory. This means that the quantity of estradiol directly links back to our ability to make, keep, and recall memories.

The same is true for the receptors in the areas of the brain that are involved in memory—both memory loss and retention. These receptors are located in the front part of the brain. They have extensions, though, that send and receive messages to and from the part of the brain where communication happens. As estrogen levels drop during perimenopause and menopause, the number of these extensions (receptors) decreases, and with it, some of a woman's recall ability.

Short-term memory loss and recall problems are bad enough, but that's not all a woman has to deal with at this time of life. Mood swings, anxiety, depression…all are equally common. All are equally signs and symptoms of dementia, too. So, you can see why Joan isn't the only one who hits the panic button. That's scary stuff! For this reason alone, it is important for us to get comfortable in talking about menopause. Knowing you aren't alone and knowing these problems are part of the experience of perimenopause and menopause are extremely important for a number of reasons; namely, the peace of mind that once a woman gets to the other side of menopause, her memory begins to improve right along with the decrease in those awful hot flashes.

That's great news, but until you are there, it doesn't do you much good, does it? And let's be honest—a woman in this condition wants one thing and one thing only—relief.

Often times their chosen method of relief is hormone replacement therapy. HRT, as it is sometimes called, is nothing more than taking estrogen, which can be delivered in several forms including cream, gel, patch, or in a tablet. To say it so matter-of-factly makes it sound completely logical. Replacing something that is so beneficial? Why not!

As it turns out, HRT isn't as cut and dried as you might think it is. Hormone replacement therapy has been linked to heart attacks and strokes. This fact is often enough to scare a woman away from HRT, but as with everything else, you need to take the time to weigh the benefits against the risks. The first and most important factor is age. Most women between the age of 40 and 60 are excellent candidates for HRT. Women over the age of 60, however, in my opinion, are not. Here's why: studies prove that women who start HRT after age 60 are between 15% and 38% more likely to get Alzheimer's.

When you combine that with the fact that Alzheimer's and most other forms of dementia strike after age 60, it's easy to see the combination of the two is not wise. The risks are not what I, or most people would consider worth taking. But for women in their 40s and 50s, without associated health risks, the benefits may be worth the risks, since the risks are minimal.

HRT is not your only option—no matter how old you are. There are several other things you can do to help yourself think more clearly.

#1: Don't stress about it. I know that one is easier said than done, but it's worth the effort. Trust me. You have to believe and rest on the truth that menopausal memory issues are not an indication of where you are headed. BUT…since two-thirds of all individuals with Alzheimer's are women, it's hard not to ignore the estrogen 'thing'. You just have to learn how to not obsess over it.

#2: Increase your physical activity. The benefits stemming from increased physical exercise are many and all of them matter greatly. You reduce the chances of obesity, which reduces the chances of diseases like diabetes. You also reduce the strain on your heart, which in turn increases blood flow to the brain. And you know what the brain does, don't you? Makes, stores, and recalls…MEMORIES!

Exercise also stimulates the release of endorphins, which are chemicals that improve your mood and prevent anxiety and depression from creeping in. Exercise also wears you out (in a good way) so that you enjoy a better quality of sleep.

#3: Consider making some changes in your diet. Make sure you are eating well-balanced meals, avoiding excessive sugar, and limiting your consumption of alcohol. For a woman, the recommendation is that they have no more than four alcoholic beverages a week. Tobacco and illicit drugs should be avoided completely.

Another dietary change you might want to consider is the addition to phytoestrogens. Phytoestrogens are a type of natural estrogen. They are found in foods like flaxseed soybeans and edamame, dried fruits, sesame seeds, garlic, peaches and berries, wheat bran, and even tofu. Cauliflower, broccoli, and Brussel sprouts are good sources, too. FYI: the research on how effective phytoestrogens are in helping with the negative effects of menopause is not well documented, but my opinion is that it can't possibly hurt, so why not? These foods are all good for you for a variety of reasons, so it's a win-win.

#4: Stimulate your brain using a variety of methods each and every day. Stimulating your brain isn't just about multi-tasking, enjoying a fulfilling career, or staying busy. Stimulating your brain happens when you:

- Learn something new
- Practice and perfect new skills
- Reading and book clubs
- Engage in conversation

- Challenge your brain with puzzles, trivia, word games, and so forth
- Coloring books, paint-by-number, and other arts and crafts
- Gardening
- Caring for a pet
- Volunteering
- Limit your screen time

#5: Talk about it. Share your thoughts and feelings about what you are going through with a few close family members and friends. Going through perimenopause or menopause is incredibly stressful. A woman needs a few peers in her corner to encourage her, assure her, hold her accountable for taking care of herself, and cheering her on. These things, along with the reminder that she is not alone can make all the difference in the world.

REMEMBER

Just remember that perimenopause and menopause cause memory issues. So, if you are a woman coming to this phase of life and have a family history of Alzheimer's or some other type of dementia, do not let these temporary issues fuel your anxiety and fear. Remember that this is a transient period of time, so take control by doing the things we've just talked about, so that you can be a happier, healthier, more confident you.

When They Forget Their Words

My wife would laugh and say something like, "Give me the thingamajig or the whatever you call it." You could tell from the look on her face that she was trying to find the right word, but just couldn't. At that stage of her dementia, she would usually 'find' the word a little later and say it, followed by, "That's what I couldn't think of earlier." Then later on, as things got worse, she wouldn't even try to figure it out. She'd just point and say, "I need that," or "May I have those, please?"

Marilyn was always such a vivacious, energetic person, yet humble, too. She was never too proud to laugh at herself when she did something silly or admit when she'd made a mistake. But I knew it really bothered her to not have the right words. The worst for her, I think, was to forget people's names. She was such a people person. Hospitality was a God-given talent for her. So, it was really hard to watch that ability slip away and know there was nothing I could do to stop it.

Mercifully, she had a stroke and died before she slipped into the darkest stages of dementia. It's been five years and I still miss her. You don't give someone 55 years of love and life and it just stop. But I know this is better for her, for the kids, and for me. For her to be here physically, but not know us—that would be far worse. ~Don

The subject matter for this chapter is something I chose to write about because of an encounter I had with my mom literally earlier today. As I've already mentioned, mom lives with us. She has her own apartment and is basically independent. Theoretically we could coexist and never see each other, but that's not the way it is. She has her own entrance, but our residences are connected through a stairwell and she comes up frequently and visits with us and vice versa.

Today was a day for one of those visits, because my oldest daughter came over with her husband, and their precious new baby. When they arrived, I called my mom and invited her to come upstairs so she could enjoy some cuddle time with our new granddaughter and great-granddaughter.

Of course mom said yes, grabbed her camera, and came right up. It was special and fun having four generations of us there together. everyone together. But after a short time, Mom started getting nervous. I started noticing this in her a couple of years ago, but lately it's been getting worse. What was once 'reserved' for large gatherings or among people she didn't know very well, is now something she struggles with even among close family members.

This nervousness I'm talking about is a level of anxiety associated with dementia that comes from having difficulty keeping up with a conversation. Her ability to recall or find the right words to insert into the conversation is declining rapidly. She doesn't understand why she can't find her words, but she knows she can't and it's unsettling. Feeling unsettled makes her nervous and feeling nervous causes anxiety. It's a vicious cycle that just keeps spinning faster and faster. And the faster it spins, the worse she gets…and feels.

It was really obvious while the kids were here—both her inability to find the words she wanted, and her anxiety over it. Bless her heart, she couldn't even carry on a conversation without struggling for words. After a while, it became more about the word she couldn't get than the word she was saying, even though she was able to participate in the conversation to a much greater extent that she thought she was. In other words, she was focusing on what was missing instead of what wasn't. It broke my heart to see her like that, but since we're all aware of the situation, none of us said anything about it or even acted like anything was amiss.

After the kids left, my mom and I ended up going for a short drive to run some errands. I didn't say anything about her having a hard time finding her words while we were gushing over the baby, but she did. She said, "I hate this."

"What do you hate?" I asked.

She said she hated having to struggle to find the words she was looking for. Even trying to say that was a struggle for her, and she knew it. She also said she felt stupid.

"Mom, this has nothing to do with your intelligence. This is sadly just part of the process," I explained. I then went on to tell her how anxiety makes the situation even more difficult. FYI: We've had this conversation before…more than a few times. But just like all those other times, in her mind, this was the first. So, we talked about it some more. I explained that the harder she tried to find that word, the harder it would be for her to find it.

I wanted so much to find a way to help her understand, and then it came to me. I told her it was like being on a diet. "As soon as you know you're on a diet you become hungry—really hungry. You want things that you've never even thought about wanting. Every commercial seems to be about food, every conversation about a meal or a new recipe you should try, or something else related to food. And all because now you're on a diet."

I then went on to explain that the same thing happens with anxiety. Anxiety over not being able to find your words only makes word-finding more difficult regardless of whether or not the person is also dealing with any sort of memory impairment. But if you do have some sort of memory impairment, when you can't find your words, you get even more anxious because you are afraid your memory is failing even faster than you thought it was, and that makes you more anxious, and that makes it harder to find your words, and on and on it goes.

"So, what do I do?" she asked. "How do you think I should handle this?"

I told her, and I'm telling you now, that the first thing I would do is try not to be bothered by it. I know that seems impossible or even ridiculous because if someone said that to me, I would probably say something like, "That's easy for you to say.". But the reality is that you don't want to fixate on the words you can't find because it's just going to be a perfect setup for forgetting yet another, and then another. Next, if you or your loved one forgets a word, just keep talking past it. People will figure out what you want to say by the context of the conversation.

I am often asked if there's a medication that can fix this. Or if anxiety medication would help. My answer to that is that I think that should not be the first option. Treating someone with medication for anxiety so that they're relaxed and calm, but not a catatonic blob that sits and stares at the wall is not always easy to accomplish. Besides, you don't want to destroy or hide someone's personality behind a drug-induced stupor, and quite honestly, that's what some medications do.

By and large, the best way to deal with this situation is to do one of two things:

1: Do what we do most of the time—nothing. Just ignore it and act like nothing is wrong. Which is actually true. Nothing is wrong. It's just part of the dementia process.

2: Offer a little help by saying something like, "Are you thinking about _____?" and offer the word you believe the word you believe they are looking for, but only if they are noticeably bothered by it.

Regardless of what you decide to do, you need to make sure your loved one knows you have their back, that it really is no big deal, and that they have nothing to feel embarrassed or ashamed about. It's really not a big deal. There are a lot worse things in life than not having the right word at the right time. You also need to remember that the less you make of it, the easier it will be for them to relax and realize it's not worth getting anxious over.

When is it Time for Hospice

Calling on hospice makes a bold statement. It says you know the end is near. It says you are ready to be selfless by letting your loved die with dignity and in peace, instead of fighting a losing battle for your sake. I know because I was at that point. But God took care of it for me, instead.

Granny had Alzheimer's and I spent seven years taking care of her throughout it all. It's not something I ever thought I would be capable of doing, but I did it and I consider it an honor and a blessing to have done so. But as Granny got worse and worse, even though I know we will spend eternity in heaven together, I wasn't quite ready to let her go. So, every time she would say something about wishing God would take her (which she did numerous times each day), I would say, I know, but I still want you here with me.

Now mind you, I was in my fifties and she was in her nineties, but I meant it—I really wasn't ready to let her go. But in the last few months of her life, she was incredibly weak and weary, and she looked so sad. One day I asked her if she wanted to sit outside or stay in and listen to some music. She said, "Neither. I want to go to sleep and not wake up until I get to heaven."

I knew right then it was time to let her go. I hugged her and kissed her and said, "Then that's what we'll both ask God to do." After that she didn't look so sad. She looked...relieved...ready.

Two weeks later, on my fifty-second birthday, I was curled up beside her in her bed when she took her last breath.

Realizing it was her last breath took my breath away—for a moment. But then I realized that giving her the peace to die was the best way I could show my love and gratitude for all she'd done for me. ~Darla

Have you ever wondered if you should call hospice, or when to know it is time to do so?

Among those who care for a loved one with dementia, or those who realize they are in the early stages of dementia, this is a conversation that should be had, but one that rarely takes place. And I think the primary reason for this, is the misconception so many people have about hospice. Specifically, what it is and what it isn't.

First of all, we need to clarify that there are two types of hospice. One that happens in a hospital or in a facility. The other takes place in the home. We are going to focus on in-home hospice, which is hospice care that allows the patient to remain in their home, while the hospice caregiver comes to them.

That statement automatically leads to the next question, which is, what does it really mean to have hospice caregivers come to your home, and what do they do?

That's a two-part question, so we will answer it that way, as well.

First, let's make sure we understand what hospice is and is not.

Hospice is NOT a means of accelerating a person's death or giving medication to cause death. Hospice IS a way of approaching end of life so that it allows the person to spend their last days, weeks, months, or sometimes even years in as much comfort as possible and with a sense of dignity.

It's not just about the patient, though. Hospice is based on the concept of treating the entire family, not just the person with the terminal diagnosis.

I have to be honest with you. I'm always a bit uncomfortable bringing up hospice with a patient's family members if we don't already have a healthy rapport. And I've already had to do it twice this week. What makes it so awkward is that I don't have any reference point to start with in knowing how they feel about hospice. I don't know whether they are open to the possibility, whether they have valid concerns about it, or if they view it as giving up.

In both situations it quickly became clear to me that the patient's needs far exceeded the family's capabilities to care for them. Not because they didn't want to, but because of the state of dementia their loved ones were in. And since it is a terminal illness, vs. a progressively debilitating illness, hospice was an option. It was an option because in order for someone to qualify for hospice, with a diagnosis of Alzheimer's or some other type of dementia, there needs to be a reasonable expectation that that person may pass within the next six months or less. Again, it's an expectation, based on the rate of progression, but it's not an absolute.

But you ask, what happens if someone signs on for hospice in six months comes in the person is doing okay? Answer: They're not discharged from hospice. We know that dementia is progressive and irreversible, so they would just go ahead and recertify that person and continue on with hospice. From an official or 'by the rules' standpoint, my understanding is that a patient must speak six words or less in the day (not counting repeated usages of 'yes' and 'no'), before being accepted into hospice. But again, there is a lot of flexibility in this. The 'big picture' is taken into consideration before making such a decision. For example, if someone is still somewhat talkative, but has no control of their bowels and bladder, or has no concept of where they are or who they are with, they would still qualify for hospice care.

The next question families usually ask is why. Why should we call hospice?

There are a number of reasons I encourage families to call upon hospice care. First of all, as I've already told you, the goal of hospice is to provide dignity and comfort for your loved one, above all else. Once someone has been accepted into hospice, their resources are limitless. If they need a hospital bed, it's provided. If they need a wheelchair, it's delivered to their home. If they have need for frequent nurse visits, they will be given and they will also have a social worker who becomes involved, as well. All their medications related to their admitting diagnosis are covered under hospice care and if you desire pastoral care, but don't have a minister you feel you can call upon, they will provide that, too. Some hospice care organizations provide transportation to and from doctor's appointments, and some even offer the options of music and/or massage therapy. And best of all (in my opinion), some hospice organizations offer respite care to the caregiver. If only for a few hours a week, the caregiver can take some much-needed and much-deserved time off without having to worry about their loved one. They know that when they leave them in the care of a hospice worker, they will be safe and will receive the utmost in care and attention.

So you see? I wasn't exaggerating when I said hospice takes the entire family and wraps their arms around them.

They understand that your loved one is not going through this alone. They understand the impact is felt throughout the entire family. That is why after your loved one passes away grief counseling is available. They don't just leave you and act as if nothing happened.

Getting back to the fundamentals of hospice, I want to reiterate that it is not a method of expediting death. But you do need to know that they are not proponents of aggressively treating terminal conditions. For example, if your loved one has dementia, and is diagnosed with cancer, they do not support chemo or radiation treatments unless it provides comfort and relief of pain. For example, if a tumor is causing pain or other issues because it is pressing against a vital organ or other body part, then palliative radiation would be covered under hospice care. That being said, if your loved one is on hospice, and they develop something like pneumonia or a urinary tract infection, and you feel it needs to be treated, which in hospice it typically would not be, you can sign your loved one off hospice temporarily, without worrying about the ability to get them back into hospice care later on.

I know this is a lot to take in. That is why I have tried to give you enough information without overwhelming you. And if you were the family member of one of my patients, I would strongly suggest meeting with hospice to talk, listen, ask questions, and get all the information you possibly can to get all the information you can, so that you can make the most informed and best decision you can for your loved one and your family.

More often than not, people choose hospice care. I've had several family members tell me it's a 'no brainer' after they see and hear what hospice really is, and the knowledge, compassion, and resources they have to offer. Words like 'relief', 'godsend', and 'blessing' are among those I hear the most from families after they have a consultation with their local hospice care workers.

If your loved one qualifies for hospice, the decision is up to you. They will not pressure you or try to persuade you to choose a care plan you are not comfortable with. They will also not try to make you feel guilty for needing help, or make you feel like you are failing your loved one. That is not what hospice is about. Hospice is about helping you help your loved one live and die with dignity.

Closing Thoughts

Dementia—arguably the worst disease plaguing the human race. I believe it's fair to say that it's the pandemic that isn't being talked about often enough. I also want to say in that my experience in dealing with both the patients and their families that dementia's devastating blows can sucker punch an entire family, bringing them to their knees (literally and figuratively speaking). But it doesn't have to be that way. Gone are the days when dementia is grounds for locking someone up and throwing away the key. Thankfully, we now live in a society that no longer believes dementia patients are expendable…disposable…nonessential. We know that dementia patients are deserving of our compassion, our care, our love, and our respect.

I hope the topics addressed in this book will be helpful to you as you go through the journey of dementia with your loved one. I hope that in reading this you now feel better informed, more adequately equipped, and know that you are not alone—that there are people like me and resources ready, willing, and able to help you and your loved one enjoy the best possible quality of life.

Made in the USA
Columbia, SC
15 November 2020

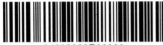